Entering the Age of Elegance

Entering the Age of Elegance

A Rite of Passage and Practical Guide
for the Modern Maturing Woman

Chloe Jon Paul

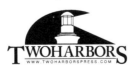

Copyright © 2009 by Chloe Jon Paul. All rights reserved.

Two Harbors Press
212 3rd Avenue North, Suite 570
Minneapolis, MN 55401
612.455.2293
www.TwoHarborsPress.com

All rights reserved. No part of this publication may be reproduced, stored in a retrieval system, or transmitted, in any form or by any means, electronic, mechanical, photocopying, recording, or otherwise, without the written prior permission of the author.

ISBN - 978-1-935097-05-1
ISBN - 1-935097-05-9
LCCN - 2008911363

Book sales for North America and international:
Itasca Books, 3501 Highway 100 South, Suite 220
Minneapolis, MN 55416
Phone: 952.345.4488 (toll free 1.800.901.3480)
Fax: 952.920.0541; email to orders@itascabooks.com

Cover Design by Wes Moore
Typeset by Tiffany Laschinger

Printed in the United States of America

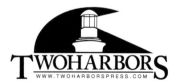

Table of Contents

Acknowledgement	ix
Foreword	xi

Part 1

Planning that Fabulous Journey	**15**
The Rite of Passage	15
How This Book Came To Be	16
Welcome to the Club	18
Let's Take Inventory	19
Dispel Those Myths about Aging	20
To Lift or Not to Lift?	20
Classy or Cheesy?	21
To Dye or Not to Dye?	24

Part 2

Entry Requirements: Staying Healthy	**27**
Your Physical Self	27
Your Emotional Self	30
Your Mental Self	49
Your Spiritual Self	52

Part 3

Luggage Check: The Relationships Roulette Wheel	**59**
SWDM: So What Definitely Matters?	59
Family Matters: The 10 Commandments of Aging Motherhood	60
The Never-Married Woman: Facts vs. Fallacies	61
Still Married: Loving It or Hating It?	62
Meeting Someone New: Pitfalls & Pit Stops	64
The Will and Grace Scenario	65
Considering a Younger Man?	66
The Older Woman and Lesbianism	66
Warning: It May Be Toxic!	68

v

Part 4
Traveler's Advisory: Managing Change and Loss   69
    Hidden Side of Change   69
    Inevitable Losses   71
    Care giving: Catastrophe or Celebration?   72
    The Experience of Grief   74

Part 5
Currency Considerations: A Mini-Guide on Practical Matters   77
    Does Money Make You Mean?   77
    What Kind of Stool Are You Sitting On?   79
    Meet Ms. Money   79
    What Is Your Estate-Planning I.Q.?   79
    Keep Your Eye on the Three Wise Men   81
    Insurance: A Quick Overview   81
    Suddenly a Widow: 9 Contacts You Need to Make   82
    Bargain or Wallet-Buster?   84
    More Savvy Shopping Strategies   84
    Household Innovations for the Elegant Woman   85
    Organized Elegance   85
    Entertaining with Style   86
    Multi-tasking in the Kitchen: A Practical How-To   87
    Bag It! Crate it! Put It in a Basket!   88
    Files You Shouldn't Be Without   91
    Recycle! Recycle!   91

Part 6
At the Boarding Gate   93
    Lost Your Zest? Get It Back!   93
    You as the Lebenskunstler   95
    Do You Have a Ya-Ya Sisterhood?   95
    Are You a Recess Girl?   95
    Meek Little Lamb or Roaring Lioness?   96

Are You a Gutsy Woman Traveler?	96
Calling All Gorgeous Grandmas!	98
Musings by Mekis	99
When Was the Last Time?	100
A Little Zest Quiz	100
A To Do List Worth Doing	101
Please Remember Me!	101
Find a Need and Fill It	102
How About a Senior-Friendly Volunteer Vacation?	103
Think MSN	105
You as a Mentor	105
Become a Mommy Mentor Partner	106
Beyond Support Pantyhose	106
Just Heard It Through the Grapevine!	108

Part 7
Ready to Fly?   **115**

A Little Homework Assignment	115
Carefully Chosen Words	116
Frank Kaiser on Older Women	116
Last Minute Details	118
Check Your Luggage	118
Your Itinerary	118
Print Out Your Boarding Pass	119
Your Passport	119

Litany of Elegance	120
Elegance Showcase: 20 WOW Women	121
Epilogue: After All Is Said and Done	123
Bibliography	125
Other Media Sources	129

Acknowledgement

My heartfelt thanks go out to the many wonderful people who encouraged me to write this book: the women (and men!) who saw its potential and timeliness.

The author wishes to thank Ruth H. Jacobs, Pamela Blair, Dotsie Bregel, and Alessa Giampaolo in a special way for their exquisite help in reading the book proposal, the manuscript, and editing. Special thanks go also to Helene Mekis, Mary Jo Sierco, Katie Desjardins, and Dr. Dorree Lynn.

To all the lovely women who shared their thoughts, experiences, and special knowledge: Thank you! May you all enjoy life's choicest blessings as you continue your journey into the Age of Elegance.

Foreword

When Chloe Jon Paul first told me she was writing this book, I thought it might be interesting. However, I was totally unprepared for the in-depth, thoughtful coverage that is both pragmatic as well as personal. I found myself surprisingly absorbed by the journey that I was invited to go on.

Entering The Age of Elegance offers so many complete luggage sets for the journey any modern maturing woman must take that it's equivalent to entering the best boutique and selecting your perfectly matched set of information for yourself. The beauty of the structure is that although it is written as a linear journey from preplanning to reaching your final destination, you can pick it up at any juncture and find a relevant gem.

I particularly like the way Chloe combines sound research with practical advice as well as wisdom culled from her own experience. She takes the rite of passage of later years seriously and obviously wants women over forty to take it seriously as well. Thus, she offers an extraordinarily detailed roadmap—better than any found on most travel guides or even Map Quest.

Upon turning fifty, I too, sought help with my new transition. As a psychologist, I also wanted to help guide my age mates with knowledge I had gleaned. I believed my purpose in life was to educate, mentor and hopefully in the process leave a legacy. Thus, I founded the online e-zine www.FiftyandFurthermore.com. Although I had fellow travelers writing on the site, sometimes I still felt alone in my journey. However, upon reading this book, I knew I had found a fellow traveling companion who could be friend, mentor and a genuine person to simply hang out with and talk. And, if I couldn't always meet her in person, all I had to do was open one of her generously shared, carefully labeled suitcases and know that I was not alone.

In this day and age of too fast everything, the art of gracious giving is too often overlooked. Entering The Age of Elegance is a generous gift to anyone who picks it up. Whether one gravitates to big picture concepts or fine line drawings, there is something special for you. Each chapter is filled with layer upon layer of information; rather like opening multiple jewel boxes nested within each other, each containing a jewel of value. As I opened each carefully selected travel case, I felt blessed with surprise gifts.

As Chloe Jon Paul begins and ends in her Litany of Elegance: "Blessed is the woman who affirms herself each day… Blessed is the woman who zeroes in on the qualities that will help her become… A Woman of Elegance," I'll add: Blessed is the woman who reads this book.

~ Dr. Dorree Lynn, Psychologist, Author, Lecturer,
   Founder/Editor-in-Chief of www.FiftyandFurthermore.com

*In loving memory of my grandmothers,
Theresa Giampaolo and Rose Buscaglia,
who gave me my first taste of elegance as a little girl.*

❧ *Part I* ❧

Planning that Fabulous Journey

Elegance: good taste, refined grace and richness; luxury free from coarseness; choiceness, refinement, grace and beauty in movement, appearance, manners.

~ adapted from the Thorndike Barnhart Dictionary and Roget's Thesaurus

The Age of Elegance denotes that period of a woman's life also known as Second Adulthood. Every woman who reaches the age of forty has the opportunity to welcome and embrace the opportunity to move into this time period with style and grace.

While elegance is not restricted to a particular age group since there are many young women who exhibit elegance, it is the older woman who can exemplify what it means to age elegantly.

The Rite of Passage

Entering the Age of Elegance is your rite of passage. It has been said that when rites of passage are not done properly, people become disoriented and lose their way in life's journey because these rites of passage are an important part of human development. Without them, one's life map is incomplete.

You are entering a new stage of life with a new identity. By engaging in a rite of passage, you enter into a spiritual experience that helps you access that which provides inspiration and guidance

Anthropologists refer to rites of passage as a liminal state which means transitional or middle phase. You are, in effect, in a condition of being neither "here nor there" at the moment but this is where transformation begins to take place. This suspended state is between past and future identities. In the first phase, which is described as separation, your old status is erased in preparation for a new one. The final phase, known as integration, you will emerge with a new social role in society.

It is normal to have heightened emotions during this time of important change in your life. That is why I'm inviting you to participate in your own personal rite of passage into your Age of Elegance.

Now let's talk about you, the debutante. Yes, this is your debut, your "coming out" time. The French word debuter means "to begin".

Of course, you are familiar with the original purpose of debutante balls or cotillions in affluent society when a young woman of seventeen or eighteen was introduced to society as being eligible for marriage. This ritual has changed somewhat in recent times but one thing has not changed. The debutante wears a white gown. Pastel shades are tolerated but it is strictly taboo to wear black or loud colors.

Now why do I mention this? It's because of what follows in this book.

How This Book Came To Be

While writing this book, I was inspired to present information in a format similar to the travel guides published by Fodor, Frommer, and Lonely Planet. These travel guides give up-to-the-minute information on how to plan your itinerary, what to pack, things to do, restaurant and hotel reviews, plus ratings for attractions of historical interest as well as photo opportunities. They even rate attractions that are "kid-friendly". They also offer advice from knowledgeable travel experts.

My philosophy of life is simple: find a need and fill it. This book is meant to be a gift to you, as you stand on the threshold of the Age of Elegance.

There is already a magnificent potpourri of books on aging but what you will find within these pages is your own personal road map for a journey into what should and can be the most exciting time of your life.

The idea for this book came about as a result of many conversations with women forty and older who really have no clue as to who they are. They have spent their lives being someone's daughter, wife, mother, or a career woman with no identity outside her profession. Now, as they approach this phase of their lives, many of them desperately want to hang on to their youth while others succumb to aging the wrong way.

Use this book to help you:
- Establish your priorities
- Investigate your options
- Zero in on the qualities that will help you become… a woman of elegance.

In the course of writing this book, I have talked with many women, and sad to say, many women cannot begin to fathom themselves as being "elegant". Yet every woman has the potential to become an elegant woman. It begins with a serious examination of self to re-discover who you really are at this point in your life. Then you can go on to identify the qualities that you already have that are attributes of elegance, refine or eliminate any behavior that might prevent you from being totally elegant, and affirm yourself as a woman of elegance.

A year ago, I tapped the wisdom of a sixteen year-old friend, Katie to hear her thoughts on aging and this is what she had to say:

It's true that I am only a sixteen year old girl but as I look ahead in my life, I cannot wait until the time when I become a crone. In the stages of life in a woman, all are important: the bride, the mother, and the crone. With each stage come important lessons and accomplishments, but aging is a beautiful process and one that should be looked forward to.

As I look at the older women in my life, I see the grace, beauty, knowledge, and experience that I can only hope to gain. I simply roll my eyes when they complain about how old they've become, and how many wrinkles and grey hairs they have. They are the most beautiful embodiment of women. They have only to reach out their hands and grasp the acceptance. They can tell stories of life because they've experienced it, and that teaching is an integral part of any young woman's life. Who better to teach you than Grandma? Mine taught me how to read, and I can only imagine someday being a grandmother and having my grandchildren learning to read in my lap.

17

> *I look forward to imparting my wisdom onto the world. I look forward to the grace and beauty that only an older woman can have. Aging is a beautiful thing.*

There is nothing ordinary about you, my dear. Too many women suffer from low self-esteem. My ardent wish for you is that after you complete this rite of passage, you will be able to look into the mirror, smile, and say, "Yes, I AM elegant!"

The first thing to remember is that elegance has nothing to do with facial features or body size. Some of the most elegant women I know are buxom but beautiful in how they present themselves to the world around them. And that's what it's all about - how you present yourself to the world around you - not just with your physical appearance but with all the components that make up the definition of elegance.

This book also offers you a practical guide for moving into the Age of Elegance. You will find some quick, easy-to-read tips to whet your appetite to read more on the subject of aging well and elegantly. Think of this book as your entry point for exploring other literature listed in the Check It Out sections and bibliography.

Welcome to the Club

Yes! It has happened whether you like it or not. So take a deep breath and step forward. You are crossing the threshold into the Age of Elegance.

You may not have had too much time to think about this momentous transition in your life until now. After all, you've been extremely busy with family, career; perhaps furthering your education. Who has time to think about "growing old"? Who really wants to think about growing old?

Then one day it hit you like a bombshell! You look into the mirror and notice the lines in your face, a strand of grey hair that you're tempted to pluck out, and you say to yourself, "Where has the time gone? Wasn't I just thirty-five?"

William DeFoore, PhD., president of the Institute for Personal and Professional Development, explains aging most eloquently in his audio CD program, *Elegant Aging: Growing Deeper, Stronger and Wiser in Your Years*: "Elegant aging is truly a matter of body, mind, emotion, and spirit. When we pay loving attention to those four aspects of our being, we age with elegance and grace."

He encourages readers to use the challenges of aging to become like the oak tree – deeper and stronger with each passing year.

So, welcome to the club! You are now part of a world-wide sisterhood; a force to be reckoned with. You have been invited to join these women who are celebrating this time in their lives.

As you journey through the pages that follow you will identify the qualities that comprise an elegant woman. You will either discover what you need to work on to improve your perspective or you will be confident in the knowledge that you're already doing it.

Let's Take Inventory

Transition: the act of passing from one state or place to the next; an event that results in a transformation passage; becoming; indicates movement, shift, change, development, metamorphosis.

Antonyms: sameness, stagnation

Think about the times you've prepared to go on a trip or to move to a new location. Packing that suitcase for a cross-country trip or even abroad required some practical thinking and perhaps a bit of ingenuity as well. You undoubtedly found ways to pack essentials efficiently, even leaving some room for items you would purchase during your trip.

Moving to a new location required a good deal of analytical thinking. What can I get rid of? How will this piece look in the new place? How did I manage to accumulate so much clutter? In essence, both situations allowed you to take an inventory: What do I consider essential? What would be excess baggage?

Now you are about to take another kind of inventory in order to answer the question: Who am I?

- What are my greatest strengths at this point in my life?
- What do I consider my greatest weakness?
- What abilities do I have that can translate into a new and meaningful experience?
- What do I need in my relationships?
- Where am I - physically, spiritually, and emotionally?
- What is one thing I've always wanted to do and haven't done yet?
- What is my Attitude I.Q.?
- How resourceful am I?
- How well do I handle change? Loss?

Answering these questions is no easy task. It requires absolute honesty and a hefty dose of humility - but hey! you can do it.

I suggest that you tackle each question through journaling. If you take a few minutes each day for the next ten days to answer one question at a time, you will have prepared your personal road map for the exciting journey you are now embarking upon.

Dispel Those Myths about Aging

Are you ready to help dispel those awful myths about aging? The media and Hollywood especially, have been selling women a blatant pack of lies about their bodies. While pharmaceutical companies and cosmetics manufacturers are laughing all the way to the bank, countless women engage in pointless anguish and self-hatred over their bodies.

What inner voice are you listening to? When you look into the mirror, are you tuned in to a positive or negative frequency?

How is it that a woman with crow's feet is considered to be a fading beauty while a man with the same crow's feet is defined as distinguished?

To Lift or Not to Lift?

Face-lifts, Botox, and liposuction are promoted as products to retard the physical aging process; in essence, they are used as weapons of denial but how healthy is it to live in denial of a life process? It is up to women themselves to change attitudes toward the older woman, and that begins with you. Like Susie Orbach, leading psychotherapist, author, and lecturer, we should be able to say, "This is who I am and I like me!"

Hollywood, especially, would have us believe that we only have a shelf life of or thirty years; thus promoting the idea that defying age via surgery is your only salvation. Aging, I repeat, is a life process and regardless of how many face-lifts a woman might have, this process continues internally as well as externally. Growing older does not have to be synonymous with failing sexual, intellectual, or emotional powers.

Your attitude toward yourself - not the retardation of the physical aging process - is what will help you age gracefully. This is a decision you must make now. Challenge those negative inner voices that fuel feelings of low self-esteem and self-worth. Your healthy acceptance of growing older starts with these issues.

A recent survey conducted by Frank About Women, a Winston-Salem, North Carolina- based strategic consultant firm, found that 66% of women over thirty-five are not afraid of aging. Only 12% said that looking younger defines aging well. The majority of women (56%) saw "aging well" as great no matter what age they are. Looking great, therefore, does not mean "looking younger".

While this study certainly doesn't reflect nation-wide attitudes because of the sampling size, it is encouraging to know that there is a group of women out there who choose to defy the myths of aging.

Classy or Cheesy?

Many women think of elegance in terms of designer clothes but Mrs. Folorunso Alakja, the former president of Fashion Designers of Algeria, doesn't equate fashion consciousness with elegance or class. She emphasizes the importance of how a woman walks, talks, and sits. Mrs. Alakja says that while she prefers to wear clothes that can make her look 10 years younger, there is no way she would want her tummy showing or cleavage as low as that of a teenager. For her, moral values, etiquette, and poise are what make a woman elegant – not expensive clothes.

Echoing those same thoughts, Karla Davis, a Florida home staging specialist, expands even further in her e-zine article, *How to be Classy and Elegant without Money*, Davis offers these suggestions:

- Smile because it creates a more pleasant environment for those around you and lifts your spirits as well.
- Learn how to take a compliment. A classy lady can do it just as well as the Oscar winners.
- Replace yelling and ranting with a calm request that exudes softness and grace. Nobody likes a fishwife.
- Answer the phone like you would if a hunk was calling. Answering in an exasperated tone of voice or one that warns the caller that she has called at a bad time is hardly elegant.
- Profanity is a no-no. Classy women do not swear and sound like a drunken sailor.
- Celebrate at a party but don't get drunk. A classy woman knows her limits and can easily mingle with the crowd sipping some sparkling water.
- Speak eloquently. There is no need to speak slang.

- Hold your head up high and walk gracefully. Classy women always appear as though they have just landed in Paris and are only in town for two days to grace you with their presence.

Timothy Gunn, fashion guru and author of *A Guide to Quality, Taste & Style,* didn't mince words when appearing on *Oprah*. His advice to the over-40 crowd was never to wear:

- Horizontal stripes
- Jackets that hit at mid-length
- Pleated pants
- Low-rise jeans
- Capri-length pants
- Double-breasted blazer

What you wear around the house is one thing; what you wear in public is another. Walk the streets of any major city and you're sure to see some pretty pitiful sights – teeny bopper wannabes.

Nancy Redd, a writer for the AOL Internet network says:" getting older doesn't mean that you have to dress like you've got a date with the nearest nursing home, but the cut and style of your clothing and accessories should be different from that of your 20-year- old hipster niece." Redd's list of "Awful After Fifty" includes: sleeveless clothing, super-low V necklines, too many strands, rings, pins, and other shiny things, hair scrunchies, grubby sneakers, and big, cheap purses.

Kathleen Tessaro, the author of the novel *Elegance,* was inspired to write the book after reading Madame. Genevieve Antoin Dariaux's *Manual of Elegance*. In an interview with Harper Collins Publishers, Tessaro gave some very solid advice. "Confidence, a sense of humor, and a lust for life make a woman attractive. A beautiful woman who takes herself too seriously or who is constantly obsessed with her looks to the point where she cannot be at ease in her own life cannot be attractive to those around her very quickly." As she says in her novel, "It's in the moments when we forget ourselves entirely that we are at our most attractive."

Now what about all those media commercials and ads that you are bombarded with? The anti-aging industry seems to be doing a booming business but I think the jury is still on just how risky or beneficial they are.

The industry now pulls in $56B a year and it is estimated that it could grow to $79B by 2009.

Did you know that -?
- More than 1500 doctors sought board certification in anti-aging medicine in 1996? A regimen of vitamins, supplements, and injections of human growth hormone (HGH) can cost up to $10K a year
- It is illegal for anyone to distribute HGH for anti-aging purposes
- Since anti-aging is not a disease, not much expense is covered by insurance
- HGH can promote tumor growth, increase blood pressure and blood clots, and cause structural damage in hands and feet
- There is no firm scientific proof that any anti-aging regimen actually slows down or reduces the aging process
- A face lift can cost as much as $20K and it takes as long as two weeks to recover
- Botox treatments cost $300 to $600 and need to be repeated every 3 to 4 months
- The International Society of Cosmetogynecology promotes plastic surgery as an extension of gynecology
- A licensed M.D. can train for as little as three days to do liposuction and injectables
- Rinoplasty, face lifts and eyebrow procedures are the most commonly botched
- Any work done on the lower face will age more quickly than on the upper face
- Several studies in the mid-1990s revealed that women choosing to have breast implants were 2 to 3 times more likely to commit suicide
- Medical tourism(going abroad to have surgery) can be hazardous with no chance of filing a malpractice suit
- Silicone breast implants have to be replaced every ten years
- The expense for initial surgery, 4 MRIs to check for signs of implant rupture and replacement surgery for breast implants runs between $11,000 and $16,000 every 10 years

- A face lift done on sun-damaged skin won't last very long and may result in more scarring
- The American Board of Laser Surgery certifies nurses and oral surgeons in laser surgery through a take-home written exam

There are many non-surgical procedures and a host of products known as cosmeceuticals. The ingredients in these products include peptides, retinoids, glycolic acids and antioxidants. Dermatologists claim that these ingredients can inhibit certain muscle movements that cause wrinkles, smooth skin tone, offset sun damage, and promote collagen production. In 2005, women spent $6.4B on these anti-aging products.

Note: Try checking out the ingredients for such products at your local drugstore and compare them to their fancy department store counterpart. You will most likely find the same ingredients at a much less expensive price. Mark Mandell-Brown, a plastic surgeon based in Cincinnati, Ohio cautions that there is no correlation between price and efficacy.

Believe it or not: There are women who use Preparation H around their eyes to reduce wrinkles. Unlike the American brand, the Canadian version of Preparation H Cream contains Bio-Dyne, also known as LYCD –Live Yeast Cell Derivative. A word-of-mouth endorsement from persons using the site www.only-in-canada.com is the only advertising you will see.

While there has been a decline in face-lifts (a 22 percent decline from 2000 to 2006), there have been 3.8M Botox treatments and 1M chemical peels. L.A. plastic surgeon Brian Kinney predicts that "all these people doing injections [now] are going to be doing face-lifts 10 years from now." While we're on the subject of Botox, horror stories abound. Just do a Google search on the Internet and you can find out for yourself.

You should, of course, protect your skin. Topical antioxidants like vitamin C or E can improve skin appearance by neutralizing free radicals that break down skin cells and exacerbate wrinkles. Retinoids, which are vitamin A derivatives, also help remove dead cells for smoother skin. They also stimulate collagen production for smoother skin. It is important to note that the data on the effects of products containing these ingredients is limited and clinical trials aren't required.

To Dye or Not to Dye?

In an interview with AOL coach Caroline Howard, Anne Kreamer, author of *Going Gray: What I Learned About Beauty, Sex, Work, Motherhood, Authenticity & Everything Else That Really Matters* stated :"Gray hair color is a very vocal symbol of 'I acknowledge who I am and I'm happy about it.' " She noted that the decision not to dye her hair was an entry to other points of self-discovery. An AOL poll taken with over 96,000 votes recorded revealed that 69% saw her as a "confident, sexy lady".

Kreamer goes on to say that the answer to that question lies within you and how accepting you are of the "seasonal changes" in your life. Most women identify with an age when they felt they looked their best – in their 20s or 30s. She notes that a century ago, life expectancy for a woman in the U.S. was only 47; now it's 80+ so we are witnessing aging like never before. Home hair coloring was introduced back in the 1950s, a time when women began joining the workforce in large numbers. The advent of easy, inexpensive, and safe hair coloring gave women a sense of "liberation" and today a majority of women dye their hair.

For years I had dyed my hair and then one day when I was in my late 50s, I looked in the mirror and asked myself: "Who are you trying to impress? Enough is enough! You have no one to impress but yourself." My hair was thinning and the dye made it even more noticeable. I decided to get a GI-Jane haircut and let the grey take over. Within a short period of time, my hair got thicker and the bald spots disappeared.

Having lived alone for several years, I wasn't exactly looking to grab any man's attention but I was soon being pursued by four different admirers who liked my classy "silver threads."

Once again, it's all a matter of choice and what feels right for you. Personally, I would rather spend my money on vacation travel. Instead of succumbing to media hype on staying "forever young", I have preferred riding a camel in the desert sands of Egypt, breaking out into a dance on the Great Wall of China, and playing with kangaroos in Australia's Great Outback. That's how I like to spend my money.

The bottom line is this: you don't need to look young in order to feel young. We might do well to heed the advice of the Dalai Lama who, while in New York, was interviewed by an AARP reporter. When asked how he felt about getting older, the Dalai Lama, then 70, replied: "I think people need to be more realistic about age. Sometimes there is too much emphasis on appearance and the artificial. Trying to look or act younger than you are is silly, very silly. The more realistic you are, the happier you'll be."

Feeling young has nothing to do with "acting young". An ever-youthful spirit engages in playfulness, seeks the opportunity to learn something new; delights in new adventures. She doesn't zone out in front of the TV or close herself off to the world around her. It is with this attitude that she not only ages gracefully, but actually relishes and embraces this period in her life.

Author Mariah Burton Nelson, also executive director of the American Association for Physical Activity and Recreation, redefines aging as a path to liberation which she calls Aging Up so that it is no longer associated with ugliness or shame. She refers to ageism as gerontophobia, saying that the term sounds like a giant dinosaur that whispers in our ear saying: "Old is ugly. Old is shameful. Whatever you do, don't look or act old." She joins the ranks of us women who strive to be authentic. Here are some of her thoughts:

Trying to look young: "It's not wrong - it's a personal choice- but I believe it's misguided. In my view, it's never healthy to try to be someone or something you're not."

Cosmetic surgery: "It's physically dangerous. People die from it each year - and it's even more dangerous to our self-esteem."

On youth being inherently more attractive than age: "Youth is not inherently more attractive than age. We just believe it because of ageism - the way some people used to believe that white skin or European facial features were 'inherently' more attractive than dark skin or African/Caribbean/Asian/Latino or Native American features."

As you ponder your decision to defy media hype and dispel those myths about aging, you may want to reflect on that great feminist Betty Freidan's approach to aging. She said that by locking ourselves into an obsession with the youth culture, we can only develop age rage and dehumanize ourselves. By giving up the denial of age and deciding to age consciously, one can continue to grow and become aware of new capacities that develop while aging.

So here's to celebrating your authentic self. Go for it!

❦ *Part 2* ❦

**Entry Requirements:
Staying Healthy**

Your Physical Self

The Basics

Turn on the TV at any hour of any given day and you're likely to be bombarded with a series of pharmaceutical commercials advertising their remedies for just about every ailment known to man. As you enter the Age of Elegance, I invite you to explore some basic, simple measures you can take to improve your physical health and reduce your dependency on pharmaceutical medication. Unfortunately, we live in a quick-fix society - pop a pill and make it better - now!

    There are, of course, life-threatening illnesses that require medication and they should be taken as prescribed by your doctor. What we're talking about here are common ailments and conditions that can be treated by using alternative methods. It takes a willingness to investigate and research what is available but more importantly, it demands discipline and consistency in establishing a regimen on a daily basis.

A word of caution: as with anything else regarding your physical well-being, always consult your doctor. Herbal supplements, when taken improperly can also create problems for you.

Is There an Alternate Route?

For years I suffered from clinical depression. I was hospitalized twice and put on suicide watch in a locked ward. Doctors told me that I would have to be on Prozac for the rest of my life "Yeah, right!" I thought, "When pigs fly!" I knew that depression results from a lack of serotonin in the brain. Serotonin is a hormone and neurotransmitter involved in sending messages through the nervous system to the brain. It contributes to mood and emotional well-being. I figured there had to be another solution for raising the serotonin level so I did some research and discovered 5HTP.

5-HTP (5-Hydroxytryptophan) is an extract of Griffonia Simplicifolia seeds from costal West Africa. 5-HTP is the direct metabolic precursor of Serotonin and is important for the production of melatonin. This amino acid has been researched since the 1970s and found to be equal to traditional antidepressants in treating depression.

I began taking 100 mg of 5HTP along with a combination tablet of calcium-zinc-magnesium at bedtime several years ago. Within a couple of weeks there was a noticeable difference. I can honestly say that I have not experienced any major depression since I've been on this regimen. Does that mean that I never have a "down" day? Of course not. We all experience a "down in the dumps' day now and then. Experiencing sadness from time to time is normal. What is important is being able to distinguish sadness from depression.

So now let me tell you about my battle with cholesterol. In spite of adhering to a low-fat diet, avoiding red meat and fried foods plus getting plenty of exercise, my cholesterol level was quite high. My doctor suggested medication which I politely refused. Once again, I searched for an alternate method to deal with the problem and found a trio of supplements that really work - gugalipid, flush-free niacin, and garlic. When blood tests were done six months later, there was a noticeable drop in my cholesterol levels. My doctor's comment was simply: "Well, keep doing what you're doing."

The Nitty-Gritty on Ultrametabolism

You've heard it all before… diet and exercise But there's a new way to look at both. Maintaining healthy eating habits is essential to aging well. We're hearing a lot about ultra-metabolism these days. There is a substantial amount of literature that gives in-depth information but I'll simply highlight a few major points. Ultra-metabolism essentially deals with weight loss. According to Dr Mark Hyman, author of *Ultrametabolism*, "By learning to work with our bodies instead of against them, we can ignite the natural fat-burning furnaces that lie dormant within us." By eating the right foods, our bodies can be programmed to automatically burn fat and keep weight off for good based on our genetic needs. He says that what we eat directly determines the genetic messages our bodies receive and these messages control all the molecules that constitute our metabolism, telling the body to store or burn calories. In his book, Dr. Hyman develops seven keys to this new science of weight loss and provides an excellent guide on how to customize the Ultra-Metabolism plan to fit your own genetic needs.

Our bodies have a natural detoxification system that eliminates waste products and environmental toxins but with today's lifestyle, that system needs more rest and support in order to keep functioning normally. In order to combat environmental toxins and the harmful effects of processed foods, too much sugar, and saturated fats, our bodies spend, in Dr. Hyman's words, "enormous metabolic capital on detoxification." He suggests undertaking a detoxification program one to three times a year. By answering the questionnaire in the book you can determine what your specific needs are.

Toxic Overload

When the organs in our bodies that do the work of detoxification are overworked, they, too, "go on strike". The result is inefficient channeling of nutrients, toxin overload, and the onset of disease. Here are some major points to consider:

Bad diet and constipation are the chief causes of toxic overload. Other sources of toxins include antibiotics, other drugs, lack of exercise, pesticides, smog, smoke, lead, mercury (dental fillings), and stress. Parasites should also be considered. Such infections are more common than most people think. Overloading your liver, kidneys, and colon with toxins can result in serious health problem. Fasting for two or three days once a month can help rejuvenate your digestive and cleansing system. If, however, you feel that your health might be compromised in some way, check with your doctor.

Lynn Hinderliter, CN, LDN, also known as Vitamin Lady on the Internet, underscores what has already been mentioned, adding that "Fasting and detoxification go together hand in hand." She notes that "until modern times, fasting was part of all religious life" and how many religious precepts were actually based on maintaining the health of the believer. To read her complete article on fasting and detoxification, log on to www.vitaminlady.com/articles/detoxfasting.asp.

Many of us are familiar with references to fasting both in the Old and New Testaments. Likewise, there is Ramadan, observed by Muslims, during which time nothing is eaten or drunk between sunrise and sunset.

Change Your "Oil Filter"

Another approach to detoxification is a body cleansing program that takes roughly two weeks to complete. There are a number of body cleansing products that can be found at your local health food store or on the Internet. I personally do a body cleansing program at the start of each season.

A good analogy is this: If we spend the time and money to change the oil and filter on our cars every 3,000 miles to keep them running efficiently, doesn't it make sense to do some preventive maintenance on our bodies as well? One writer likens the state of a body needing detoxification to a city where sanitation workers have gone on strike. When garbage piles up on curbsides and if the strike were to continue, it would result in a crisis leading to disease and probably an epidemic.

Chronic Pain Relief

Pete Egoscue, anatomical physiologist, who operates the Egoscue Method Clinic in San Diego, offers an exercise therapy program to treat musculoskeletal pain. He has taught women this method to achieve permanent chronic pain relief without pain medication, physical therapy, or surgery. He emphasizes that addressing your health and well-being by counting years is a mistake. While age may be implicated in many illnesses, he says he doesn't know of a single disease that is actually caused by age.

It all boils down to metabolic efficiency which means you have to get moving to keep those joints and muscles working to capacity. Arthritis worsens with immobility. Brisk walking and gentle yoga are two methods to incorporate into your action plan.

So what is your action plan going to be? What physical health improvements would you like to make? Investigate options that can work best for you and remember: continuity is the key.

Your Emotional Self

The word emotion can evoke a wide assortment of feelings we experience. These feelings can be positive or negative and as long as you are a living, breathing human being, you are bound to experience most of them in a lifetime.

The elegant woman will choose to deal with her emotions in a way that will not forfeit her dignity and serenity. While this book is not intended to explore a full range of emotions, we'll take a look at a few of the more common ones you're likely to experience at this time of your life. We'll also explore some remedies you may find useful.

John Mayer, PhD., a University of New Hampshire psychologist and Peter Sclovey, PhD., a psychologist at Yale University first coined the phrase "emotional intelligence" in the late 1980s. They proposed that "emotional intelligence" - intelligence inspired by strong emotions - might mean the difference between making an ordinary decision and a creative one.

Later, Daniel Goleman obtained their permission to use the phrase "emotional intelligence" and expanded the concept to produce the 1995 best-selling book with that phrase as its title. Goleman reasons that we have, in a sense, two brains, two minds, and consequently two different kinds of intelligence because the amygdali and prefrontal lobes of the brain are responsible for emotional response. The neocortex and other limbic structures, he explains, are responsible for rational thinking.

Goleman describes five domains that constitute emotional intelligence:

- **Self-awareness:** Being able to recognize a feeling as it is happening is crucial. The inability to recognize these feelings makes us feel overwhelmed.

- **Managing emotions:** Life is bound to be a rough ride at times. Having the ability to bounce back quickly from an upsetting situation rests upon the extent of our self-awareness.

- **Recognizing the emotions of others:** This is where "people skills" come into play. The ability to "tune in" to the emotions of others suggests developing a good deal of empathy.

- **Self-motivation:** Whether it's a short-term or long-term goal, we must have the ability to monitor our emotions so that they don't interfere in the pursuit of that goal.

- **Handling relationships:** A person may be brilliant academically and produce innovative ideas but if she is lacking in interpersonal effectiveness because of her inability to manage the emotions of others, then not much will be accomplished.

In a sense, emotional intelligence may be even more important than I.Q. because true success in life cannot be achieved without it. While there are no validated tests to measure emotional intelligence, there are a couple of versions that can be used just for fun to see how you measure up.

Check It Out
- www.eihaygroup.com
- www.ihhp.com
- www.testcafe.com
- www.allthetests.com
- www.us.mindmediacentraltest.com

The Stress Factor: How Do You Rate?

While stress is a natural part of life, the elegant woman will choose NOT to make it her way of life. She will make use of some simple, practical tools to manage her stress when it occurs. Amy Scholten, MPH, and former writer for Healthgate Data Corporation, designed a stress questionnaire comprised of 25 statements. Three possible answers: most of the time, some of the time, and rarely are given point values. A score interpretation of the respondent's stress level is given as a general assessment. The stress scale ranges from 25 to 200. Having a score between 25 and 50 means that you're doing an excellent job of managing stress but look out if your score is above 150! The questionnaire appears online at www.beliefnet.com/healthandhealing/stresscenter. Scholten notes that a more in-depth assessment ought to be obtained from one's mental health care provider. Physical symptoms of stress include headache, racing heart, cold hands or feet, trouble sleeping, and frequent colds.

If she wants to age gracefully, the elegant woman will understand the importance of managing her stress life wisely. Scientists have identified a direct link between aging and stress. A pioneer study published in 2004 was the first to confirm that chronic stress speeds up the shriveling of the tips of the bundles of genes inside the cells. This, in turn, shortens the life span of those cells, causing them to deteriorate. There is a stress hormone, cortical, which weakens muscles, causes skin to wrinkle, impairs hearing and eyesight, diminishes cognitive ability, and ultimately causes organs to fail.

Marcus Padulchick, author, lecturer, and consultant, developed 101 ways to cope with stress. If you log on to http://www.marcuspadulchickcom, you'll find his list. Here are a few of my personal favorites from that list:

- Laugh out loud without worrying about what the neighbors think.
- There is nothing more cathartic than a good belly laugh in the privacy of your home.

- Stand in the rain with your mouth open and taste the raindrops with your tongue.
- Sing out loud; sing in the shower - just sing!
- Dance -alone or with a partner.
- Get a massage.
- Say 10 nice things about yourself each morning in the mirror.
- Take a hot bath with candles and soothing music.
- Plan a "retreat day" in your home.
- Notice where there is tension in your body - imagine that body part melting like an ice cube.

Don't allow stress to force you into a corner of emotional paralysis because once that happens, it's hard to break free. Many older women find themselves on the brink of emotional paralysis especially when decisions have to be made. Generally, these decisions revolve around caregiver issues, finances, or having to deal with change and loss.

It is at such times that speaking with a counselor is most beneficial. A good licensed clinical social worker can be just as effective (maybe even more) than a psychiatrist. When physical symptoms arise that suggest a disorder, we pick up the phone to call the doctor. Why not do the same when we're feeling poorly on the emotional level?

So…Have Your Pity Party!

Is it bonafide depression or temporary sadness? Of course there will be sadness now and then. Learning to tell the difference between depression and sadness requires a bit of soul-searching.

As I said already, we all have a down-in-the-dumps day now and then. It is only when the major symptoms of clinical depression are persistent over a lengthy period that a doctor's evaluation is in order.

Having a bout with the blues entitles you to having a "pity party" that should last no more than an hour in duration. Set your alarm or kitchen timer to monitor the time and when the bell or buzzer sounds, simply say aloud: "Okay, pity party's over! Time to move on!" Crazy as it sounds, it really works!

If your "blue mood" has been caused by a person, your mantra could be: "Sorry - you can't live rent-free in my head. No vacancy!"

If the blues creep up on you because of a certain situation, make up your own mantra or say something like: "I am a strong woman and loveable." Repetition throughout the day is not only desirable but necessary. Play some upbeat music throughout the day or read a joke book to help you out of your rut.

Learning to Affirm Yourself

Self-affirmation is a healthy ingredient for a stable emotional life. I personally advocate looking at yourself in the mirror each morning, winking, and saying to yourself aloud: "Hey kid, you're okay!" Posting a statement on your refrigerator door is another way of reminding yourself of just how special you are. To negate your good qualities is nothing more than false humility which isn't worth a damn!

Someone once compared affirmations to Feng Shui, saying that they can provide "cures" to the stuck energy in our lives. Feng Shui is the Chinese practice of placement and arrangement of space to achieve harmony with the environment. By placing and arranging those affirmations in strategic spots, you will eventually experience an inner harmony.

Joan Sotkin, entrepreneur and author, say that our thoughts, beliefs, and emotions (TBEs) create our reality. The quality and nature of TBEs determine the actual course of our lives. If you have been programmed to think negatively most of your life, it will take some time to turn things around but the good news is that it can be done. Once you've identified the negative emotion that may have been long buried in your sub-conscious yet causes you to act out in the present, you can create an affirmation to release that emotion. Sotkin gives a good example. If you experienced disappointment in childhood, you may find yourself often disappointed in the present. You can say: "I release my need for disappointment". This, she says, "will help stimulate your subconscious to help you understand your need which will lead to a change in behavior." For more information, log on to www.prosperityplace.com

Learning from Emotional Pain

Buddhism explains how pain can be a great spiritual teacher. Pema Chodron, an American Buddhist nun, talks about recognizing the need "to relax into the pain" not avoiding the place that makes one feel bad, unacceptable, or unloved. She says that in her own case, resistance to the idea that she was unlovable only made the pain worse so she advises to 'turn toward the pain' [because] avoidance of pain keeps us locked in a cycle of suffering."

In order to understand this concept more fully, I strongly recommend her best-selling book, *When Things Fall Apart*. It is a must-read for anyone experiencing emotional pain.

The FGA Quotient

In the vast spectrum of emotions, there are three that appear to be most common in relation to aging. The elegant woman is not exempt from having to deal with these negative emotions. What sets her apart is the manner in which she chooses to deal with them.

So… what is your FGA quotient? FGA refers to frustration, guilt, and anger. These three emotions top the list for older women.

The first order of business is to make friends with frustration. It will show up, like an uninvited guest no matter what. How you handle it is entirely up to you and how you perceive it. There are the daily minor frustrations that tempt us to lose patience with ourselves and others. It may be a glitch in the computer program you're working on, or a telephone call from a loved one whose demands haven't been met; or having to clean up a mess you didn't make.

Then there are the mounting frustrations often associated with long-term care giving. You may be caring for a spouse, an elderly parent, or even a grandchild. These frustrations are real and potentially harmful not only to your emotional health but your physical well-being also. It is essential to identify what is at the core of your frustration and to develop an action plan to work through it. You can be proactive instead of being reactive. Think about the tone of voice you use, certain gestures you make, the kind of language you use in such situations. The woman of elegance is in control of these things and will exude a refined calmness in the most frustrating circumstances.

The second emotional hurdle to jump is guilt. Too often, at this stage of life, we find ourselves saying "I could've, I would've, I should've if only…"

The elegant woman gives herself permission to make mistakes because she accepts herself as a fallible human being. She also knows that every mistake is a perfect opportunity for learning.

Guilt is actually a good thing because it alerts us to the fact that our behavior needs to be corrected. It's the voice of our conscience telling us that something needs to be resolved. Unresolved guilt is bad because it can lead to mental health problems and disrupted relationships. Living in a guilt cycle can also be hazardous to your health. To acknowledge your feelings is to get to the core of what makes you feel guilty. That will help break the guilt cycle. Then try re-labeling the guilt that you feel. For example, instead of saying "I feel guilty about not visiting Mom more often" try saying "It would be nice if I could manage to visit Mom more often."

You might also try substituting "I feel sad…" or "I regret…" This should help you be more understanding of how you feel, what you do, and the situation you find yourself in.

The third component of the FGA quotient is anger. No one is exempt from this emotion. Our anger may be rational or irrational but everyone experiences it to some degree because it is a natural response to pain or hurt. The Woman of Elegance will look for constructive ways to deal with her anger because she values her dignity and serenity.

Since anger is a secondary emotion, the primary emotion that triggers it must be identified and dealt with. Anger is to your emotional system as a fever is to your physical system. It is a symptom of a deeper problem.

You can choose to look at anger in three different ways:
1. It is wrong, destructive, and harmful
2. Whether you suppress anger or express it violently, it causes damage.
3. Anger can be beneficial and bring about positive results.

If you make a conscious decision to take a stand on dealing with your anger, it means that you are willing to take a good, hard look at what is really making you angry, develop some tools to communicate more effectively, and try a bit of creative problem-solving techniques.

Someone once said that anger shuts out the humanity of the other person. It fosters the desire to hurt that other person. You can, however, find ways to use anger with honesty and channel it into something good.

You may even want to try some exercises to deal with anger. A personal favorite of mine is the Sacred Anger Exercise, described by Marajen Moore in her article "Exploring Anger as an Ally". It can be found on her web site http://www.awaken to life.net.

Another excellent source to help you deal with your anger is Dr. William DeFoore's web site: http://www.angermanagementresource.com. Here you can take a quick anger test and check out twelve anger management techniques.

Frederick Beuchner, a Presbyterian minister and American author, probably sums it up the best:

> *Of the seven deadly sins, anger is probably the most fun. To lick your wounds, to smack your lips over grievances long past, to roll over your tongue the prospect of bitter confrontations yet to come, to savor to the last toothsome morsel both the pain you are given and the pain you are giving back - in many ways it is a feast fit for a king. The chief drawback is that what you are wolfing down is yourself. The skeleton at the feast is you. (Taken from www.wisdomquotes.com)*

There are plenty of books that deal with anger management so the focus here is simply a gentle reminder to get you started in addressing the issue if it pertains to you so that you can move more gracefully into the Age of Elegance.

The F-Word You Need to Use

Now that you have examined anger and how it may be affecting your life, the next logical step is to check out where you stand on forgiveness. Yes, that's the F-word you must learn to put into practice. We forgive - not necessarily because that person deserves to be forgiven - but because it frees us up. In essence, you are taking back your power.

When we hold on to some resentment, grudge, or hatred toward someone, we are actually empowering them. It certainly isn't bothering that person. As Dale Carnegie once said: "Our enemies would dance with joy if they knew how they were worrying us…" (taken from www.quotedb.com/quotes851).

Experts tell us that the inability to forgive is a serious self-transgression because it exists solely in the self and doesn't impact at all on the other person for whom it is intended. Dwelling on past hurts simply does not benefit you in the present.

Learning to forgive isn't easy but seeking revenge still identifies you as the victim. Process your anger or your grief so that you can be more receptive to the act of forgiving. Being able to forgive requires courage and compassion. It may help to read inspirational stories of forgiveness or log on to a web site that focuses on forgiveness. You may need the help of a therapist but just remember this: forgiveness is for you. As long as you hold on to the pain, you remain bitter. Letting go will make you better.

Now you might say: "Well, I can forgive but I can't forget." It is true that forgiveness doesn't obliterate what happened. Remembering the hurt has us believe that we can build a protective wall around ourselves to make sure that we don't get hurt again. Unfortunately, it doesn't work out that way. All we wind up doing is adding a thick, crusty layer of bitterness over a heart that longs to be free.

In the Lord's Prayer, which is recited by Christians world-wide, we hear these words: "Forgive us our trespasses as we forgive those who trespass against us." Those words offer food for thought - and action. The Jewish tradition of atonement, Yom Kippur, is a day of reflection to seek the forgiveness of God and others as well as coming to terms with the decision to forgive those who have caused harm or pain in one's life.

Forgiving Yourself

As you enter the Age of Elegance, there are probably moments when you look back on your life and wince with pain over some of the mistakes you've made - mistakes for which you haven't forgiven yourself.

As a former lead facilitator for the Alternatives to Violence Project, an international conflict resolution program, I conducted prison and community workshops. One of the exercises in the AVP manual focuses on forgiveness of oneself. There are four questions posed in this exercise:

1. What would you have to give up in order to forgive yourself?
2. What would you lose if you did?
3. What blocks forgiveness for you?
4. What could a friend say or do to help you find forgiveness?

You might try answering these questions in written form. Another tool you might want to try is the 4R's guideline that some relationship experts recommend:

- **Regret:** Do you genuinely regret the action or hurt you've caused?
- **Repentance:** Have you offered an apology?
- **Restitution:** Did you try to find a way of making it up to that person?
- **Rehabilitation:** Have you made an honest effort not to repeat the mistake again?

In conclusion, consider this quote by Paul Boese, a well-known TV producer: "Forgiveness does not change the past, but it does enlarge the future."(taken from www.Quoteland.com).

Emotions Anonymous - It Really Does Exist!

Emotions Anonymous was founded in 1971 in St. Paul, MN. At present, there are over 1200 chapters in 38 countries. EA is not a medical or psychiatric service, nor does it provide counseling. Group meetings, which are online as well as at different locations, are held with a rotating leadership which facilitates the meetings.

EA is similar to Alcoholics Anonymous with a 12-step program. It also includes the 12 Traditions which are guidelines for members, concepts, the Serenity prayer, and EA literature. Weekly meetings, telephone and personal contacts are available.

This group emphasizes that it is not a sounding board for continually reviewing one's miseries but a way to learn how to detach oneself from them. While it considers itself to be a spiritual program, it doesn't advocate any particular belief system. The 12 Steps do, however, suggest a belief in one's higher Power. Religion, politics, national and international issues are not discussed.

EA respects anonymity, aiming for an atmosphere of love and understanding. The only requirement for membership is for one to commit to become emotionally healthy. For more information, visit their web site at www.emotionsanonymous.org.

So What Are You Afraid Of?

Fear is legitimate and necessary because it alerts us to danger and harm. Out-of-control fear, however, paralyzes you and can turn out to be a self-fulfilling prophecy.

What do aging women fear? There are ten common fears most older women have so take a good look at each one and see if it applies to you.

1. **Growing older and more feeble**

You have already experienced hard times physically and emotionally but you've survived, haven't you? The good news is that experts tell us that 80% of the population over 65 is doing just fine. These persons are functional and independent. You can maintain strength and agility with proper diet and exercise, Walk, stretch, bend as much as possible everyday and see what a difference it makes.

2. **Being alone**

Being alone does not have to mean being lonely. More women are living alone today by choice than ever before. Florence Falk, author of *On My Own*, says: "Aloneness is an opportunity, a state brimming with potentiality, with resources for renewed life – not a life sentence. Its cultivation should not be an apology but an art. In the space of aloneness – and perhaps only there- a woman is free to admit and act on her own desires. It is where we have the opportunity to discover that we are 'not a half' but a sovereign whole."

Aside from active adult 55+ communities, a growing number of Boomer women are discussing the possibility of setting up communal living arrangements with life-long friends who find themselves in the same situation. How about a pet? A dog or cat is wonderful company. I have three cats that are more affectionate than many people I know. They are attuned to my moods, wait for me at the door to greet me when I arrive home, and ask for little or nothing in return while giving me many moments of joy. Each one has a distinct personality, bringing humor and playfulness into my daily life. Pet ownership does entail some work and expense but the benefits of having a little furry companion to talk to and cuddle make it worthwhile.

3. **Being a burden**

If you don't want to be a burden to others, you had better have a plan. We generally think in terms of becoming a burden to our children but there are many older women who don't have children so there is even more reason to have a plan in the event that you become ill or disabled. I recently told my two adult children about my 5-year plan, adding that if unforeseen circumstances arise in the meantime, the plan will be re-evaluated and revised. I also had my advance directives videotaped by a professional videographer and made into DVDs for my family.

You can make things a lot easier for your family by organizing your medical, personal, financial, and legal record now. I highly recommend *The Senior Organizer* by Debby Bitticks, Lynn Benson, and Dorothy Breninger. Log on to http://www.BioBinders.com or call 800-791-8071 for more information.

4. **Pain**

Whether it is chronic or temporary, pain increases with tension and fretfulness. Explore your options for dealing with it. Being better informed about the cause and nature of your pain can actually help reduce it. Using visualization techniques (guided imagery) has been found to be very effective.

5. **Losing control**

Whether it means losing control of your mobility, certain bodily functions, or mental capacity, it's a plain fact that no one wants to be in that position. Unfortunately, we have little control over such things, especially as we age. But what about people who have been afflicted this way since childhood or even birth?

If you want to be inspired and deeply touched, read *Ten Things I Learned from Bill Porter* by Shelly Brady. It will undoubtedly re-define your thinking on losing control. Bill Porter, born with cerebral palsy, became a door-to-door salesman for the Watkins Company in Oregon. With the patience and persistence instilled in him by his mother, he became salesman of the year. A newspaper article about him resulted in a TV appearance on ABC's 20-20. The book, which was written by his assistant, was made into a movie. Now in his mid-70's, Bill takes orders for Watkins products online.

6. **Losing independence**

The freedom to come and go as you please can never be taken for granted. There may come a time, however, when you will have to rely on public transportation instead of driving your car. Granted, there are many women in their late 80s and 90s who still drive responsibly but you don't want to be like the 84 year old woman who crashed into the wall of a school cafeteria, killing an 8-year old boy.

Annual hearing and vision tests are a must. Check with your local senior center to see what they offer in the way of transportation services. If you're living in an adult retirement community, bus service to the local shopping center and mall is readily available.

Consider using bus service or metro rail for certain outings instead of driving so that if and when the day comes that you're no longer able to drive, you will be able to transition a little better.

7. **Not having enough**

Younger women complain of not having enough time to do all the things that need to be done. For older women, not having enough generally translates into lack of money or perhaps, even love.

Allianz, a Minnesota-based life insurance company, says that in a survey of about 1,925 women, a startling 90% say that they feel financially insecure. Forty-six percent of these women have a tremendous fear of becoming a "bag lady" and regret not having learned more about managing money while in school.

Jay McDonald, an MSN money columnist, describes the Bag Lady syndrome as a fear women have that their financial security could disappear in a heartbeat. If you have this particular fear, you're in good company. McDonald cites Lily Tomlin, Gloria Steinem, Shirley MacLaine and Katie Couric as harboring the same anxiety.

You can live well on less but you have to be daring enough to think outside the box. I call it "creative calculating". There are countless ways to cut down expenses. In her book, *The Next Fifty Years: A Guide for Women at Midlife and Beyond,* Pamela D. Blair, PhD. offers some excellent tips and also a gentle reminder being frugal is not the same as being cheap.

8. Abuse

Current statistics show that 4% of seniors over 65 (1M) may be abused or neglected in some way each year. Abuse can be physical or psychological. Neglect may be active or passive.

Sadly enough, there are many older women still putting up with an abusive husband. I heard one woman say recently: "We've been married for 60 years but it hasn't been all that good." I have witnessed verbal abuse tolerated by a few of my women friends over the past few years and wonder why they allow it. If you fear potential abuse or see signs of it happening, seek professional help before it gets to a crisis stage.

9. Crime

Another major fear of older women is becoming a victim of crime, and yes, it can happen in broad daylight. Break-ins, car-jacking, assault, and robbery have no age restrictions. An example of this is what happened to an older woman in a Wal-Mart parking lot in Portland, Maine.

As she was returning to her car in the early afternoon hours, a woman in her late 30s approached her asking if she could borrow her cell phone. As this older woman attempted to respond, the woman sprayed her in the face with Mace, grabbed her purse, and ran off.

Some time ago, my home was broken into during the day. Fortunately I wasn't home at the time but it left me feeling vulnerable and afraid. Needless to say, I had the locks changed immediately and an alarm system installed the next day. There are precautions you should take on a daily basis:

There are precautions you should take on a daily basis:
- Use the ATM machine only during daylight hours.
- Always lock your car - even when you're driving.
- If you suspect someone is following you, don't go home. Drive to the nearest police station.
- Never give out personal information over the phone or on the Internet.

- Keep your cell phone handy when you're alone in the car.
- If you plan to be away from your home for any period of time, make sure that you alert a neighbor.

Identity Theft, Fraud & Scams

Yes, they're all out there waiting to nab you, my dear, and they're likely to prey upon the older folks. They won't stand a chance with you because you are entering the Age of Elegance fully equipped to do battle with anyone who would dare to mess with you. Here are some quick tips and facts to store in your arsenal of self-protection:

- Mark your calendar with the dates bills are due to arrive. Identity thieves steal mail. Call the company if you suspect a bill is missing or overdue. Go over your account statements line by line. Purchase a mailbox with a lock if you live in a private home. Neighborhoods that used to be considered safe have become increasingly susceptible to crime.
- Block out you social security number on your Medicare card.
- Never carry your social security card in your wallet.
- Get a free credit report annually by calling 1-877-322-8228 or log on to www.annualcreditreport.com. The credit report should only have the accounts you are currently using. Please note that purchasing identity theft protection service is not necessary. It is already free.
- Do not sign the back of your credit card. Print "photo ID required" instead. If your card is already signed, use a whitener to remove your signature and then print over it.
- When you write a check to pay on your credit card, write the last 4 digits of your account only in the space labeled for the memo section of the check.
- Photocopy the front and back of your driver's license, credit cards, Medicare card, and passport. Put that information in a safe place.
- Don't put your phone number on your checks.

- If you do online banking, check your information frequently.
- Never allow any company to debit your account.
- Receipts should only show the last 4 digits of your credit card account.
- Check your mobile phone's serial number by keying in #06#. A fifteen digit code will appear on the screen. Write it down and store in a safe place. If your phone is stolen, call your service provider and give them this code. This may not work with pay-as-you-go phones.
- Shred-shred-shred. If you don't already have one, purchase an inexpensive shredder and shred anything containing personal information that you would ordinarily throw in the trash.

If you should become a victim of identity theft, do the following:
1. Call 1-877-IDTHEFT (1-877-438-4338).
2. File a report with the Federal Trade Commission.
3. Contact all 3 credit bureaus to place a fraud alert (see Appendix for phone numbers).
4. Close all your accounts.
5. File a police report.
6. Call the social Security fraud line at 1-800-269-0271.

Did you know that -?
- it is illegal for companies not to secure your personal information
- you can delete all the web sites you visited while online by pressing Ctrl H before logging off the Internet (You may want to check your Web browser's help file on deleting browsing history if this doesn't work for you.)
- a company called Choice Point sells your personal information but it is not considered illegal
- you can stop credit card solicitation that comes in the mail by calling 1-888-OPTOUT (1-888-567-8688)

- you can put an end to all those catalogs coming in the mail
- Send a request to :

    DMA Mail preference List
    P.O. Box 643
    Carmel, NY 10512

- you can sign up with OnGuardOnline.gov to get practical tips on how to be on guard against Internet fraud, secure your computer, and protect your personal information
- you can set up a Google Alert at www.google.com/alerts which will let you know when its "crawler" finds pages with your name
- you can reduce telemarketing calls by registering with the National Do Not Call Registry by calling 1-888-382-1222 or by logging on to www.donotcall.gov

This registration is good for five years.

- you can take precautions to insure that your charitable donation dollars really benefit the people you want to help? Check out the charity you plan to donate to at one of the following web sites:

    BBB Wise Giving Alliance: wwwgive.org
    American Institute of Philanthropy: www.charitywatch.org
    Guide Star: www.guidestar.org

- foreign crooks targeting people in the U.S. account for 45% of telemarketing fraud
- people 60 and older are especially vulnerable to magazine sales scams, sweepstakes, and phishing by phone

These are calls pretending to be from a well-known source asking you to confirm your personal information.

10. **Dying**

"Death is not extinguishing the light; it is putting out the lamp because the dawn has come."

~ author unknown

Another favorite anonymous quote on a more humorous side is:

"Everyone wants to go to heaven but nobody wants to die."

Are you so much afraid of dying as of thinking that you really haven't lived? Death is a universal transition that we are all destined to make, and since tomorrow isn't promised to anyone of us, it is essential that we live each day to the max.

As you enter the Age of Elegance, facing your own mortality can be challenging but it doesn't have to be frightening or morbid. While death is familiar to us with the passing of our loved ones and cherished friends, it raises many questions because we cling to what we can see but feel apprehensive about what we cannot see.

The Woman of Elegance recognizes that death is linked with sleep. As Shakespeare wrote: "Sleep [is] the death of each day's life..." We go to bed each night in full expectation of awakening the next day. We know that sleep is necessary in maintaining good health. Yet, there are many unanswered questions as to how we lose consciousness every night when we fall asleep - and regain it when we wake up. Consciousness is not a function of the physical body. While there is a good deal of information about "the neurology of sleep", there is no real answer to why consciousness informs the body that it must sleep.

Ingrid Van Mater states succinctly in her article "The Mystery of Death and Rebirth": "When we retire and willingly leave behind our daily consciousness, giving in to the invisible realm awaiting us, we are preparing ourselves for the more complete sleep which is death."

There are countless records of near-death and out-of-body experiences that give some insight to what comes next. Back in the mid-90's, I was a Hospice volunteer working with AIDS patients. It was my task and privilege to be a source of comfort to them in their final hours. I'll never forget Ken. Realizing that he probably had less than 48 hours to live, I said: "How's it going, Ken?" He looked at me, smiled, and replied softly: "I've got one foot in the water and it's feeling just fine."

My own personal story involves an out-of-body experience. In 2003, I attended the Monroe Institute in Faber, Virginia to learn more about the Hemi-Sync method and attaining a higher level of consciousness.

Upon our arrival for the week-long retreat, participants were told not to have any pre-conceived notions or expectations on what they would experience; that there was no assurance that we would experience anything. Each day we were individually sequestered in a cubicle surrounded by thick, black drapes and guided through a series of instructions and metamusic (which I'll explain in detail later) which we listened to using headphones while lying on a bunk.

While I didn't experience much in several sessions, I was totally unprepared for what happened in one particular session. I had the sensation of being in a high-speed elevator zooming upward with all the color of the rainbow whizzing past me until I encountered a dazzling white light which turned into a sphere. I followed the sphere as it regressed into the distance ahead only to find myself facing an incredibly beautiful crystal bridge. Then I heard a voice (my Spirit Guide?) say: "Chloe, you can play on the bridge for a while but you can't stay. You still have stuff to do." Reluctantly, I had to return to the present.

Now for some practical matters that will help lessen your fear of death:
- Do you have Advance Directives? If not, it's time to do so. Have you designated someone to hold durable power of attorney for health matters and personal property? Since this is a touchy subject, you would be wise to consult an attorney.
- Are you pre-paid? Smile if you must but this is a practical matter that can be taken care of in advance. Whether you choose cremation or traditional ground burial, this is one thing you can do to relieve your survivors of an additional burden.
- Have you thought about planning your own funeral or memorial service? This is a wonderful way to prepare for that inevitable event that awaits all of us.
- What would you like your final gift to your loved ones to be? One of the nicest things I've ever done was to make a DVD which tells the story of my life in photographs (taken from family albums which no one looks at anymore), using a music background; then followed by a taped message by me to my loved ones. It only runs 12 ½ minutes but is a complete and lasting remembrance.

Check It Out
- www.aarp.org: Planning for Incapacity: A Self-Help Guide
- www.abcd.caring.org : A Handbook for Mortals by Americans for Better Care of the Dying.
- www.compassionindying.org:

The A-B-C's of Handling Your Fears

Now that we've explored the most common fears older women have, here are some suggestions for you to consider:

- Name your fear. Say it aloud. Write it down and focus on solving the real problem – not just some small aspect of it

- Talk to yourself aloud. We talk to ourselves in the silent mode all the time. Voicing your fear aloud reduces the fear.

- Since your imagination is running wild with this fear anyway, purposely exaggerate all the bad things you think might happen. You'll discover that it's these exaggerated scenarios that you're really afraid of.

- Use your imagination in a positive way. Visualize yourself being less afraid. Breathe and exhale deeply. Better yet, imagine that you've already dealt with the fear. Mentally review how you handled it

- Make plans to confront the fear head-on, be it a thing, a person, or a situation. Planning in advance reduces the fear and increases your power to transform it into something positive.

- Above all, believe in yourself. Once you have identified your ears, you will grow more confident.

So… what are you afraid of?

Your Mental Self

As we age, our minds do change but don't be deluded into believing that stereotype which equates aging with loss of mental function. Now that you've stepped across the threshold into the Age of Elegance, you will want to spend some time investigating what you need to know about keeping your brain healthy. You have the ability to continue learning as long as you live. Although it might require more time and effort, you retain that ability if you do the things that are necessary to maintain a healthy brain.

You may find yourself processing information at a slower pace and your reaction time in responding to a situation may be slower but that is because of changes taking place in your nervous system over time. What about your memory? Perhaps you've already experienced some memory loss and you're thinking: Uh-oh! I'll bet I'm a candidate for Alzheimer's! Relax!

Memory loss can happen well before you reach 50. If you are experiencing occasional memory loss, it could be due to such conditions as stress and anxiety, depression, diabetes, B-12 deficiency, infections, and prescription drugs as well as over-the-counter drugs.

While short-term memory (less than 30 minutes) can worsen with age, long -term memory (months to years) is basically permanent. To illustrate this point, my mother, who suffered from dementia beginning in her late 80's couldn't tell you what day or year it was but could tell you the name of her fourth grade teacher.

Gary Small, MD, author of *The Memory Bible: an Innovative Strategy for Keeping Your Brain Young* states that only one-third of memory loss is genetic. That means that people have more control than they think. Ultimately, that means we have the potential to influence a large component of our brain-aging. So, what is the influence that you can have?

Brain Nutrition

It is said that your brain is the greediest organ in your body and that it requires very specific dietary requirements. Your daily intake should include: essential amino acids found in dried beans, green leafy vegetables, some animal products, whole grains, eggs, nuts, and seeds; Omega 3oils / fatty acids found in salmon, tuna, sardines, avocado, fresh coconut; antioxidants found in many fruits; beta-carotene, vitamin C and E, vitamin B-12, niacin, thiamine, potassium and magnesium.

Did you know that -?

- vitamin B-12 deficiency and thiamine deficiency are a recognized cause of impaired cognitive function

- sodium, potassium, calcium, and magnesium are key mineral ions in the brain and should be maintained in critical balance

- magnesium can reduce brain irritation and block seizures

- over 50 double-blind, placebo-controlled studies give evidence that ginkgo has beneficial effects for memory function more than any other herb

- your brain uses approximately 20% of the total oxygen pumping around your body

- your brain consists of about 100 billion neurons - about 166 times the number of people on this planet

- the speed at which your brain performs cognitive skills tends to decline after age 25

- your working memory (very short-term) stores ideas just long enough for you to understand them and can hold an average of a maximum of seven digits. Think about that the next time you look up a phone number and remember it long enough to dial

16 Tips for a Healthy Brain

1. **Physical exercise:** Research shows that people who get plenty of physical exercise can wind up with a better brain. Find a way to enjoy your exercise rather than forcing yourself to do it. Brisk walking, yoga, stretching and bending (even when you're on the phone) should be part of your routine.

2. **Brain exercise:** Rev up those inactive sections of your brain with some of the suggested activities which follow.

3. **Music:** Listen to Baroque music, Mozart, or investigate the metamusic offered by the Monroe Institute

4. **Alcohol:** Keep it to one drink a day. It's a known fact that alcohol can kill brain cells.

5. **Play:** Card game and board games give your brain a chance to think strategically.

6. **Sleep:** Need to remember something? Review the information that you need to remember. Write it down and then sleep on it. Studies show that sleeping on it increases retention 20 to 30 per cent.

7. **Track your mental state:** Our consciousness has peaks and valleys during the day. Higher consciousness lasts roughly 90 minutes with 30 minutes of low consciousness that follow. Concentrate on important mental tasks when your mind is most "awake" and work on creative tasks when you're in a state of lower consciousness.

8. **Learn:** Whether it's new vocabulary or a foreign language; taking a course at your local college, or traveling, be open to learning something new.

9. **Concentrate:** Identify what's distracting you at the moment and

decide if you need to deal with it immediately or whether you can put it on your "to do" list. It will allow you to be in a more relaxed state so you can think more clearly.

10. **Aroma therapy:** Perk up your brain with a whiff of peppermint or lemon oil. It really works!
11. **Don't stop asking why:** Your brain is wired to be curious so don't stifle that curiosity. Get in the habit of asking "why?" often.
12. **Memorize:** Whether it's your password, driver's license number, or lines of poetry, make an effort to memorize something on a regular basis.
13. **Laugh:** Your laughter releases endorphins and other powerful chemicals that help reduce stress. Think of laughter as "charging your brain's batteries".
14. **Link:** Pair a person's name with a color, sound, or action.
15. **Strategy:** Make lists categorizing your shopping, and errands. Always put your car keys in the same place.
16. **Other-Handedness:** Try brushing your teeth or writing a memo with your opposite hand to challenge your brain.

Fitness and Fun for Your Brain

The Brain Fitness Program, developed by Posit Science, is a computer-based training program which participants complete by spending one hour a day five days a week for eight weeks. The six exercises focus on auditory processing which is related to cognition. For more information, log on to www.positscience.com.

AARP's web site www.aarp.org features fun and games such as Rotonym, Word Search, Universal Trivia, Jumble, Sudoku, and Jigsaw Puzzle. This is a neat way to give your brain a mental work out for a few minutes each day.

Brain Age, inspired by the prominent Japanese neuroscientist, Dr. Ryuta Kanashima, provides quick mental activities for brain stimulation. It is played on a hand held Nintendo DS system which allows you to write your answers with a Stylus pen. The speed and accuracy of your response determine your brain age. The DS and Brain Age are sold separately and are available wherever video games and home entertainment products are sold. Happy Neuron games (www.happy-neuron.com) offer a broad spectrum of mentally challenging activities based on the five critical thinking skills: memory, attention, language, executive functions, visual and spatial memory. Games like Elephant Memory, Secret Files and Ancient Writing are fun to play and you can enjoy these games for a few pennies a day with a monthly subscription of $9.95 which can be canceled at any time. An Adobe Flash Player is required in order to play. The games were created by Drs. Michel Noir, Bernard Croisile, and Frank Tarpin-Bernard for Quixit, Inc. a US-based company.

Your brain, the command and control center that runs your life can be compared to a supercomputer weighing only three pounds. Yet it determines the kind of person you are- in how you feel, act, and respond to other people. Now, more than ever, as you enter the Age of Elegance, you will want to preserve your brain power, optimizing its function so that you can be the best that you can be.

Your Spiritual Self

Spirituality is often misconstrued as having a religious affiliation with a church, mosque, or synagogue. Nothing could be further from the truth. There are many church-going individuals who attend weekly services who are anything but spiritual. Likewise, there are many persons who follow a regimen of meditation and private prayer who wouldn't dream of entering a place of worship. The ideal can, perhaps, be found in a combination of the two. Spirituality embraces a number of other disciplines besides prayer and worship. Yoga, tai chi, reciting a mantra, chanting, and meditation are excellent channels for attaining spirituality.

Whatever your current status in this area, you have reached a time in your life when taking inventory includes looking at the spiritual you.

Medical Science and Spirituality

The acceptance of spirituality in medicine has grown. There have been over 1200 studies on the healing power of faith and the effect of spirituality on one's health. The body possesses a physiological response to repetition of a phrase or action.

Dr. Herbert Benson at Beth Israel Deaconess Medical Center in Boston, and Dr. Harold Koenig at Duke University Medical Center have led the way in discussing the power of prayer, merging spirituality and the sciences. Dr. Benson suggests that a person's belief in a Higher Power can reduce visits to doctors' offices by 35% to 50% a year. Persons who experience spirituality tend to have fewer medical symptoms.

A study led by Dr. William Strawbridge of the University of California at Berkley, which was released in 1997, tracked more than 5,000 Californians over 28 years. It revealed that people who frequently attended religious services had lower death rates, were more likely to stop smoking, had more social contacts, and stayed married longer than those who did not.

Health experts tell us that when we share our innermost thoughts with God (Higher Power, if you will), our immune system gets a boost; our brains release chemicals that serve as natural painkillers and mood enhancers. There are now 72 medical schools in the United States offering some kind of course on spirituality and healing. In December, 2006, the Harvard Medical School Department of Continuing Education and the Mind/Body Medical Institute at Beth Israel Deaconess Medical Center presented a conference called "Spirituality and Healing in Medicine: Practical Usage in Contemporary Healthcare". The emphasis was placed on showing doctors how to respond to patients' spiritual concerns in a sensitive way even though they may be pressed for time.

Dr. Christina Puchalski of George Washington University, one of the presenters at the conference introduced what she refers to as the "FICA questions" that healthcare workers can ask patients. FICA, she explained, is a mnemonic device for faith, importance, community, address. The questions healthcare workers are encouraged to ask are: Do you have a faith tradition? How important is it? Are you in a faith community? How might we address these issues in your healthcare?

Dr. Benson emphasized that translating belief in God (and 90% of Americans do believe in God) into health and well-being is not an alternative or complementary but… scientifically based and proven.

Try Some of My M & M's

No, it isn't those multi-colored chocolate coated peanuts that everybody loves. The two things that have worked wonders for me are meditation and the metamusic that I previously mentioned. That's why I refer to them as my M & M's.

Let's talk about the nuts and bolts of meditation. It is quiet thought and reflection; contemplation on sacred or solemn subjects. There are many techniques that can be used to teach your mind to become calmer and better focused. You don't need formal training to do it. Here are some simple guidelines to help you:

- **Choose a time of day.** Ideally, early morning is best. At first, you may only want to spend 10 minutes in meditation. As you progress, you can spend a longer period of time.

53

- **Choose a quiet space.** The spot should be a place where distractions are minimal. In good weather, a garden or sunroom enhances the experience.

- **Mentally voice an affirmation or intention.** Make a positive statement about the day you expect to have. For example: "Serenity will surround me throughout the day".

- **Sit in a comfortable position.** Many people sit cross-legged on the floor. This isn't essential but you may want to try it. The important thing is to assume a position that allows you to be focused. Don't lie on a bed or rug.

- **Be patient with yourself.** Your mind does not always want to focus and you may find distracting thoughts surfacing. Don't pressure yourself when this happens because it will detract from your enjoyment of the experience. With time and practice it gets better.

If you want to explore specific techniques, you can choose between Eastern (most notably Buddhist, Tao, or Zen meditation) and Western (Christian). There are several interesting web sites which offer excellent tips on meditation.

Check It Out
- www.meditainment.com
- www.higherbalance.com
- www.Chopra.com
- www.learn-to-meditate.com
- www.ananda.org
- www.meditationiseasy.com
- www.mediationcenter.com (offers a free 21-day newsletter)

Finally, let's take a look at what is NOT meditation. It is not-
- **concentration:** In meditation you don't focus on a task. You simply remain aware of the moment.
- **relaxation:** It is the outcome of meditation since the effect of calm and serenity that comes with meditation makes you relaxed.

- **religious practice:** Meditation is not necessarily connected with any specific religion or ritual.

- **state of mind:** It is said that meditation is really the state of no mind. Scientists tell us that there are four states of mind based on the frequency of brain waves. When you meditate, you are in the Alpha state where excess mental activity slows down.

- **self-hypnosis:** In meditation you don't enter into a state of semi-conscious trance the way you do in self-hypnosis. You remain in a state of consciousness with an awareness of the here-and-now.

- **thinking:** Meditation transcends the thought process. Our minds create all kinds of thoughts constantly but in the meditative state, you achieve an awareness that is independent of all kinds of thoughts.

Metamusic

Metamusic, developed by the Monroe Institute, is a combination of exquisite musical selections and the Hemi-Sync® is an audio technology based on how the brain functions naturally. It helps you safely alter your brainwaves with multi-layered patterns of sound frequencies. When listening to these sound frequencies through stereo headphones, your brain responds by producing a third "sound" (electric signal) called a binaural beat which encourages the desired brainwave activity. The CDs produced by the Monroe Institute feature many titles with special blends of the Alpha, Delta, and Theta frequencies which slow excess mental activity and facilitate meditation and relaxation. A word of caution: Never listen to metamusic while driving or using machinery. The musical selections range from New Age to timeless classical pieces. Here are just a few examples of what is offered:

- **Ascension:** features the electronic music of J.S. Epperson's "music of the spheres" and Hemi-Sync®. It promotes a state of mental calm and expanded awareness.

- **Spirit's Journey:** Composer Mark Certo's inspirational music blended with changing Hemi-Sync® signals will guide you into different states of consciousness in your journey of self-discovery.

- **Portal to Eternity:** referred to as contemplative electronic music by Dr. Micah Sadigh and Hemi-Sync®, provides a "refreshing departure" from your daily activities.

- **Special note:** Hemi-Sync® does not embed subliminal messages.
- For more information, log on to www.MonroeInstitute.org or request a catalog by calling 1-800-541-2488.

What's in Your Spiritual Pantry?

- **Books:** There are many excellent books on the market that fall under the category of spiritual reading. They can't all be listed here but I'll mention a few that I have found to be exceptionally worthwhile in my journey toward the Age of Elegance.

    - *When All You've Ever Wanted Isn't Enough* by Harold Kushner
    - *A Purpose-Driven Life* by Rick Warren
    - *Everyday Tao* by Deng Ming Dao
    - *Chicken Soup for the Soul* by Jack Canfield and Mark Victor Hansen
    - *The Seven Spiritual Laws of Success* by Deepak Chopra
    - *The Alchemist* by Paolo Coelho

- **Journaling:** Keeping a daily journal (even if you only write a couple of lines) is an excellent way to track your spiritual journey because it is here that you can articulate your deepest thoughts.

- **Silent Retreat:** Whether you go to a retreat center, monastery, or spend the day at home, you can have a day that is totally engulfed with tranquility. If you elect to do this at home, turn off the computer, telephone, radio, and TV. Immerse yourself in the stillness and watch what happens with the changes in your body's rhythm and activity of your mind.

- **Beliefnet.com:** This web site has something for everyone. The link Faiths and Practices provides information on every religion. Other links include holistic spirituality, guided meditations, healing prayers plus much more. You can even take a personality quiz by clicking on to Belief-O-Matic to identify your religious and spiritual beliefs.

So there you have it! As you enter the Age of Elegance, you can move forward with confidence to nurture your spiritual self. The Woman of Elegance seeks balance and harmony in her life.

❦ *Part 3* ❦

**Luggage Check:
The Relationships Roulette Wheel**

SWDM: So What Definitely Matters?

Whether single, widowed, divorced, or married, you are definitely part of that acronym and that means examining your relationships. As you enter the Age of Elegance, it is a good time to examine your relationships to determine which ones are toxic and which ones continue to flourish.

The Boomer Age has produced more educated, savvy women than ever before so it isn't necessary here to offer Relationships 101. Rather, here are some gentle reminders:

There will always be some measure of conflict in any relationship but you can be assertive without being aggressive.

Learn how to deliver an I-message that describes the provoking situation (you're attacking the problem - not the person); how it makes you feel and why it makes you feel that way. Try saying it without using the word you. Be specific about your needs. A typical I-message would sound like this: When _____ (describe the situation), I feel ____ (take ownership of the emotion you feel at that moment) because _____ (give the reason why you feel that way). What I need is ___. Can we talk about this now or later? You may even want to try what I like to call my "magic words": "Tell me what you need."

Learn to recognize the things that make you "go off" 80% of the time. Those "triggers" may actually be situations or events that happened to you a long time ago. When they surface, it's easy to transfer them on to what is happening at the moment.

Avoid shutting down or withdrawing. Instead, ask for some "time out"

Family Matters: The 10 Commandments of Aging Motherhood

Married, widowed, or divorced, you most likely have children and grandchildren. In today's world where more single women are opting to have children, this may be true as well. Consider these four ground rules that you can and should establish with your adult children. They should be able to:

- honor your privacy and independence.
- not make unreasonable request of time or money.
- visit and call regularly but not daily (unless you prefer it that way).
- enjoy you as a person and friend - not just as their mother.

Your grandchildren may still be toddlers or young adults at this point in your life. You will be a prime example to them of what it means to age well, gracefully, elegantly. They will learn this by what they observe in your behavior, your speech, but most of all, your attitude. You have the right to remind them of acceptable behavior when they are in your house but leave the disciplining to Mom and Dad.

And now, my dear, I ask you to consider:

The 10 Commandments of Aging Motherhood

1. Thou shalt not make unreasonable demands of your children.
2. Thou shalt not be an enabler, continuously giving hand-outs to an able-bodied adult child.
3. Thou shalt not give unwanted advice.
4. Thou shalt not "tidy up" when visiting in their homes nor overstay your welcome when visiting.

5. Thou shalt not make snide remarks about the son-in-law or daughter-in-law.
6. Thou shalt not complain about your personal problems.
7. Thou shalt not give gifts simply because you like them.
8. Thou shalt not pry into their personal lives.
9. Thou shalt not bring up painful memories in conversation.
10. Thou shalt not fret when they don't call or visit as frequently as you would like.

Remember that they have their own lives to live.

The Never-Married Woman: Facts vs. Fallacies

"People ask me about it all the time. I say, Ralph Nader never married and he's my age (62). Do you ask him the same question?"

~ Gloria Steinem, American feminist,
journalist and advocate for women's rights

The mythology surrounding the older, never-married woman is that she is lonely, longs for love, and is afraid of dying penniless. Research suggests the opposite. Studies conducted on the never-married women finds that they are happier, less lonely than people think, and have a greater sense of psychological well-being than their single male counterparts. The terms "old maid" and "spinster" no longer apply. Many never-married women have affairs and some opt for a live-in relationship. They don't hate men and aren't afraid of sex. They are simply unwilling to give up their independence or settle for a mediocre marriage. Some never-married women who find a need for children are having them out of wedlock or choosing to adopt. Others find satisfaction in nurturing nieces and nephews.

Anastasia Toufexis, a former editor at *Time* magazine notes that lifelong singles have been staging a 'quiet revolution', fighting social stigma, family pressures, and even their own misgivings to set a new model for it means to be an accomplished, fulfilled, satisfied woman.

Check It Out
- Flying Solo: Single Women in Midlife by C., Stewart, S., Anderson, & S. Divrudjan,

- The Improvised Woman: Single Women Reinventing Single Life by Marcelle Clements
- Singled Out: How Singles Are Stereotyped, Stigmatized, and Ignored and Still
- Live Happily Ever After by Bell DePaulo
- Solitaire: The Intimate Lives of Single Women by Marian Botsford Fraser
- Bachelor Girl: 100 Years of Breaking the Rules – a Social History of Living Single by Betsy Israel
- With or Without a Man: Single Women Taking Control of Their Lives by Karen Lewis
- Our Lives for Ourselves: Women Who Have Never Married by Nancy L. Peterson
- The New Single Woman by E. Kay Trimberger

Still Married: Loving It or Hating It?

You may be surprised to learn that one out of five first marriages lasts 50 years, despite what we hear about the high divorce rate. Retirement, illness, and other life changes can still put a strain on your marriage even if you have enjoyed a lasting, happy marriage.

If you are entering the Age of Elegance as a married woman, you may want to take some time to answer these questions:

- Do I share my emotions freely?
- Am I a good listener?
- Do my spouse and I talk about our sexual relationship?
- Are we attempting to rediscover one another?
- Is there anything we need to re-negotiate in our marriage?
- Do any rules have to be changed?
- Are we able to discuss finances calmly?
- Is there something new that we can learn or do together?

- Do we regularly express our contentment and appreciation for each other?
- What is my expectation of a shared workload around the house at this time in our lives?
- What do we share spiritually?
- Do we encourage each other's independence?

Ideally, these questions might be used by you and your mate to work on individually and then shared with one another.

Check It Out
- Claiming Our Deepest Desires: The Power of an Intimate Marriage by M Bridget Brennan, & Jerome L. Shen
- The 30 Secrets of Happily Married Couples by Paul W. Coleman
- Pure Gold: A Lifetime of Love and Marriage by Hugh & Ruth Downs.
- I Like Being Married: Treasured Traditions, Rituals & Stories by Tony Evans & Therese L. Borchard

If you happen to be one of the 25 million unmarried women in America, you are, hopefully also part of that 63 percent of single women living alone who see their older years as a time to transform their dreams into reality. Do you remember that zany sit-com "Golden Girls"? If you're widowed or divorced, you may be able to identify with Dorothy, Blanche, Rose, or even Sophia, Dorothy's mother. As mismatched as they appeared to be as housemates, they really cared about each other and supported one another. It was also a time for them to re-invent themselves.

And so it is with you. Whether widowed or divorced, you have the opportunity to "defy gravity" by daring to "fly" to pursue your dreams and discover your authentic self. Rev. Marsha Lehman, M.Ed., MA, a life coach, explains that there may be a discomfort in doing this because we are not used to exposing ourselves to ourselves.

In reality divorce and widowhood are much alike. The widow grieves the death of her spouse; the divorcee mourns the death of her marriage. In both cases, there is no linear timeline for the grieving process. Our grief is as individual as our lives.

Did you know that most women over fifty - ?
- don't want to remarry
- want to downsize domestically because they've "been there - done that"
- realize that "blended families" can cause all kinds of conflict
- don't need a man to support them financially

Entering the Age of Elegance means that you have grown wiser; that you are becoming more proficient in discerning your needs and wants. The Universal Law of Attraction begins to take on a special significance for you. This law, which is the most powerful force in the universe, stated simply, says that you get what you think about, whether wanted or unwanted. With this in mind, your daily mantra could be: "Today I will attract all that is good and beneficial to me."

Check It Out
- Flying Solo: Single Women in Midlife by Carol M. Anderson, et al.
- The Improvised Woman: Single Women Reinventing Single Life by Marcelle Clements
- On My Own: The Art of Being a Woman Alone by Florence Falk,
- Suddenly Single: Money Skills for Divorcees and Widows by Kerry Hannon,
- After He's Gone: A Guide for Widowed and Divorced Women by Barbara Jowell

Meeting Someone New: Pitfalls & Pit Stops

The woman who wants to date again will consider a solid blend of good timing and careful planning. The elegant woman possesses a certain confidence because she is comfortable with herself. This is reflected in her speech, her smile, her posture, her eye contact -all necessary ingredients for attracting a desirable man. If she decides to date again she knows that:

- She is emotionally ready
- It isn't wise to date within the first year of a divorce or the loss of a spouse, or partner.

- Online dating has certain advantages but common sense and caution are necessary.
- Personals ads in the classified section of the newspaper are also a possibility but can sometimes be deceptive.
- She will not mistake loneliness for love.
- She can be sexy but savvy. Before she engages in a sexual relationship, she will weigh the risk of HIV/AIDS and other STDs and ask the right questions - even request testing.

There are many places where you can meet new people casually and feel safe. Here is a sampling of places and events you can try:

- singles dances
- volunteer activities
- sporting events
- bereavement groups
- political campaigns
- book clubs
- college/adult ed groups
- church groups
- support groups

The Will and Grace Scenario

Much has been written about a platonic relationship between a man and a woman.

While it is true that certain relationships that start out as a friendship blossom into romance, relationship experts say that men and women can be good friends and that there are good reasons for them to do so. This, of course, refers to heterosexual men and women. But what about straight women and gay men? Current research suggests that heterosexual women welcome a friendship with no sexual overtones. Women feel valued for their personality and not their sexuality while gay men claim that a friendship with a heterosexual woman is very fulfilling because they can trust them and rely on them.

For over thirty years, I was fortunate to have one of the most endearing and enduring friendships with my friend Jack. Although we never openly discussed his sexual orientation(You just didn't do that back then), I suspected that he might be gay. It didn't matter because we shared each other's joys and sorrows for many years. The hugs and kisses we gave each other were familial - not sexual. My husband liked him as well. When he died a few years ago, I felt that I had lost an older brother.

Considering a Younger Man?

A recent AARP poll reveals that almost one-third of women between the ages of 40 and 69 are dating younger men. If you are considering this option, take note to some sage advice from Kathryn Elliott, Ph.D., assistant professor of psychology at the University of Louisiana at Lafayette. She suggests that the key to making such a relationship work is based on choosing someone who shares the same intensity about life as you do. This has nothing to do with age. If one partner wants to go out but the other prefers staying in; if one wants to talk, and other wants space, it is not likely to work.

Can such a relationship ever last? Will he leave you for a younger woman? If he wants children, that is a possibility. Susan Winter co-author with Felicia Briggs, of *Older Women, Younger Men: New Options for Love and Romance* interviewed more than 200 couples for their book and states that the average length of such relationships was 13 years and some couples had been together 25 years or more.

The Older Woman and Lesbianism

The older woman who is in a lesbian relationship has special needs to consider as she enters the Age of Elegance. Even though she may be living with a same-sex partner of many years, she would be wise to get her medical and financial directives in order so as to protect herself and her partner.

The older lesbian should know that it is especially important to state in writing that is notarized what her end-of-life care wishes are. The healthcare representative whom she chooses will have the power to make decisions when she is not able to. She should also indicate who can visit her if she is hospitalized and be sure that her doctor puts a copy of her request in her medical record. She should also designate someone to have financial power of attorney.

She should purchase long-term care insurance because gay and lesbian couples who share a home don't have certain protection under Medicaid laws and could risk losing everything if one of them should have to go into a long-term care facility. Fortunately, there are resources to help with these and other issues

SAGE (Senior Action in a Gay Environment) was founded in 1977. It is the nation's oldest and largest social service and advocacy organization for LGBT senior citizens. It offers individual and group counseling through its Clinical and Social Services as well as educational programs and social activities under its Community Services program. Another feature is the Caregiver Program which helps caregivers with respite care and limited financial help.

OLOC (Old Lesbians Organizing for Change) is a national organization which provides a forum for lesbians over 60 where they can come together and speak for themselves. It uses the term "old" to (as they put it) "refute the lie that it is shameful to be an 'old' woman. We will no longer accommodate ourselves to a language that implies in any way that 'old' means inferior."

OLOC holds a national gathering every two years and produces a newsletter that addresses issues of being an old lesbian. There are also local chapters that hold meetings and social gatherings.

Hot off the press: The latest edition of *A Legal Guide for Lesbian & Gay Couples* by Hayden Curry et al. Curry has partnered with other lawyers to write this book. It contains valuable information on domestic partner benefits, wills and estate planning, power of attorney, property, and contracts.

Strange but true…Relationships Australia, a non-profit counseling organization funded by both the federal and state governments is actually encouraging lonely, older single women to become lesbians. The spokesperson for the group, Jack Carney cited men's shorter life span and their pursuit of much younger women as factors that force older women to turn to other women for love and companionship.

Check It Out
Websites
- www.couple-national.org
- www.sageusa.org
- www.oloc.org.
- www.silverthreadscelebration.com

Books
- *Lesbian Passages: True Stories as Told by Women Over 40.* by Marcy Adelman, ed. Alyson Publ. 1996.
- *Lives of Our Own: Secrets of Salty Old Women* by Caroline Bird. Houghton Mifflin, 1995
- *Ageism in the Lesbian Community* by Baba Copper. The Crossing Press, 1987.

Warning: It May Be Toxic!

Unlike many household cleaning products and packs of cigarettes, toxic individuals don't have a label stamped on them that says: hazardous material... may be dangerous to your health. In an online interview with David Roberts at www.heathyplace.com, Dr. Pamela Brewer, a holistic psychotherapist, described a toxic relationship as one in which you are feeling harmed either emotionally or physically. It is one in which you are chronically tired, angry, frightened, or worried.

Why does one stay in a toxic relationship? Some of the reasons are:
- low self-esteem
- fear of being alone
- depression
- threats from the hurtful partner
- having grown up in a toxic household
- religious convictions

If you believe that you're in a toxic relationship at this point in your life, it's time to call the Poison Control Center (a good counseling service) and make plans to move on with your life. While this sounds easier said than done, it is possible once you decide to take charge of your life.

As Chuck Spezzano's book title states: *If It Hurts, It Isn't Love*. His message is simple and to the point. If you're in pain, you must have chosen something other than love. The book contains 366 principles (one for each day including Leap year) to help heal and transform your relationships.

On a final note: In her book, *Something More-Excavating Your Authentic Self*, Sara Ban Breathnach says: "Bad men are spiritual graces sent in disguise to teach us through torment to love ourselves."

Part 4

Traveler's Advisory: Managing Change and Loss

"Time isn't the enemy. Accept that nothing lasts forever and you'll start to appreciate the advantages of whatever age you are now."

~ Oprah

As you enter the Age of Elegance, you must be prepared to face change and loss. The Woman of Elegance recognizes that both are inevitable and takes proactive measures to deal with them. She knows that her ability to adapt is a reflection of her mental and emotional health. She doesn't, however, simply want to adapt; she wants to succeed!

Hidden Side of Change

Edgar Papke, CEO and president of Living Change, a Denver-based consulting firm, offers valuable insight to understanding the "hidden" side of the change process. At first glance, change and transition may seem identical but Papke differentiates between the two stating that "Change involves the actual shift in the environment; in the external situation. Transition is the internal psychological reorientation people go through in coming to terms and dealing with a change in their environment and in their lives. It involves a personal process that engages a wide range of individual emotions." Papke's writing draws on the expertise of William Bridges and his book *Managing Transitions: Making Sense of Life's Changes*. The change process which occurs in these phases has been described as:

- **The Endings Phase:** An event has occurred and your response might be shock, denial, feeling stunned. It's important to recognize your feelings and to consider all your options on how to move forward.

- **The Transitional/Neutral Phase:** This is where reality sets in and many emotions surface. It is a very intense period and requires effort in disengaging oneself from old patterns and the way things used to be. It is the time when you begin setting some new long-term goals in order to create a new future for yourself.

- **Moving On/New Beginnings Phase:** You have survived the change and you've discovered that life is still good; that you've grown. Now you are moving in a new direction with new commitments and possibilities. It's time to celebrate!

Change can be anticipated or unanticipated. Perhaps you are looking at a change of residence, career, or even lifestyle. Because these changes are anticipated, you have the luxury of time to plan ahead. Unanticipated change doesn't allow that luxury. A crisis arising from a major accident, sudden death of a loved one, or a natural disaster can happen at any time.

Carol McClelland, PhD. of Transition Dynamic Enterprises, Inc.and author of *The Seasons of Change*, presents a lovely analogy in describing change, likening it to the change of season.

During Fall, there is a sense of change on the horizon and the first order of business is to acknowledge that change is about to occur. Denial of such change should be avoided at all costs. It's important to get the support you need and to consider all your options.

In early winter, you may be experiencing fatigue and confusion so it's important to create a time of quiet and reflection for yourself. It can be a time of self-renewal. You should avoid staying too busy or starting something new until you've had enough time to analyze your situation and identify your desires.

The Winter Solstice is the experience of looking at your life from a new perspective and as McClelland compares it to drawing a line in the sand as if to say enough is enough. Creating a new story about your past may open new doors to the future. Investigate all possible solutions, avoid being in a toxic environment, and continue to provide yourself with ample quiet time.

In Late Winter, you begin to have a glimpse of new insights and you should follow them wherever they take you. As you create a plan for your future, be certain that you have a clear picture of where you want to go without moving ahead too rapidly. On the other hand, it's equally important to move out of your comfort zone and embrace the new opportunity.

Spring is a time of new growth and you begin to feel new energy. Trust your own timing to allow the birthing of what is new in your life and the blossoming of the new you. Don't be afraid to move forward.

Summer finally arrives and you will allow what is new in your life to ripen naturally as you celebrate your success.

Your perception to change determines the approach you take. You can:

- avoid it (flight)
- resist it (fight)
- harness and guide it (opportunity)

The bottom line is - people actually do love change! Think of the myriad changes that we make on a daily basis - clothes, hairstyles, furniture, jobs. Having all this experience with minor changes is really a dress rehearsal for major ones that put us on the path of a new adventure on the road of Life.

In *"Healing Words for the Body, Mind and Spirit"*, Caren Goldman says: " In meeting a challenge, we become witnesses to our ability to go where we haven't gone before, do what we've never done before, and arrive at a new place in our lives. Indeed, once witnessed, the courage, fortitude, self-trust, and even the humility that helped carry us through can never be 'unwitnessed'".

Inevitable Losses

Loss can mean the death of a loved or the ending of a meaningful relationship. It can mean having to give up treasured possessions when down-sizing in a move to a new residence. It also involves the physical deterioration of our bodies when sight, hearing, and motor ability become impaired.

Now here's the good news: you are more resilient than you think. You have had, as Betty Freidan once said:" a lifetime of practice in adapting to different roles." You will refuse to become a victim of circumstance. You will choose to find some positive meaning in what happens.

Care giving: Catastrophe or Celebration?

Countless women entering the Age of Elegance find the task of care giving suddenly thrust upon them, whether it be a spouse, an elderly parent, or even grandchildren. Oftentimes, it occurs as a result of an unforeseen crisis with little or no time to prepare for it.

The dictionary defines care as feeling interest, concern, solicitude. The word *give* means to hand over without pay, to furnish, supply, devote, dedicate, sacrifice. There is another word, however, that supersedes care giving and that word is caretaking. It means giving unconditionally while taking responsibility for nurturing oneself.

The saving graces of caretaking can be summed up in three words: humor, spirituality, and self-care.

Try to see the humor in situations that might otherwise cause frustration. Better yet, learn how to inject humor into what's happening that you may find annoying or upsetting. Case in point: One day my sister and I picked up our mom at the nursing home to take her out to lunch. Mom was suffering from a severe case of dementia so we always had to deal with repetitive questioning. That day, while in the car, it was "Where are we going?" Each time she asked, we simply repeated "to the restaurant". After the fifteenth time of "Where are we going?" my sister answered. "Ma, we're going to pick up men" - to which Mom responded enthusiastically: "Ooh! That sounds like a good idea." Surprisingly, she stopped asking about where we were going and we enjoyed a good, hearty laugh.

In terms of spirituality, my personal favorites are what I already mentioned previously - what I call my M&M's - meditation and metamusic. It's also a good idea to post significant thoughts around the house. They will uplift your spirits. Check to see what is in your "spiritual pantry". Those spiritual staples can help tide you over the rough spots. Caretakers need to be reminded that self-care isn't a luxury. It is one's right as a human being. There is no need to feel guilty so take some time to re-energize.

The Woman of Elegance will take a proactive role in turning what could be a catastrophe into a celebration because she will:

- believe in herself and trust her own judgment.

- protect her own health so that the care recipient's health is not at risk.

- reach out for help.

- develop as many creative problem-solving tools as possible.

In the final analysis, instead of saying "I could've, I should've, I would've... she'll be able to say "I did it!" And she'll be glad she did.

Check It Out
Web Sites
- www.nfcacares.org

- www.parentcare.com

- www.caregiving.com

- www.nih.gov/Alzheimers/Caregiving

- www.thefamilycaregiver.org

- www.agewiseliving.com

Books
- *Elder Rage* by Jacqueline Marcell

- *Quick Tips for Caregivers* by Marion Karpinski, RN

- *Coping with Your Difficult Older Parent* by Grace Lebow and Barbara Kane

- *Doing the Right Thing* by Roberta Satow

- *The Caregiver Survival Handbook* by Alexis Abramso

- *Minding Our Elders* by Carol Bursack

- *Caregiving and Loss* by Kenneth J. Doka and Joyce D. Davisson

- *Learning to Speak Alzheimer's* by Judith Koenig Coste

- *Daily Comforts for Caregivers* by Pat Sampler

The Experience of Grief

"Grief is the price we pay for love."

~ author unknown

As I stated earlier, our grief is as individual as our lives. While there are stages of grief, there is no linear timeline for it. As you enter the Age of Elegance, you have probably experienced it more than once already and you know that it shows itself in all aspects of your life: psychological, physical, spiritual, cognitive, and behavioral.

There are four major tasks of grief described by J. William Wordon, a well-known grief therapist who has lectured and written on topics related to illness and bereavement. He suggests that you:

- Accept the reality of the loss and realize that reunion is impossible since that the loss is irreversible.

- Work through the pain of grief and allow all your feelings to be acknowledged; seek help along the way.

- Adjust to your changed environment and make an effort to fill the void.

- Re-locate the deceased emotionally so that you can move on with life. Initially, it can be a struggle in adapting to a new role and responsibilities. You may feel unsafe and helpless. Adjustment requires time and effort but as you begin to experience new emotional energy, you can begin to cherish the memories and plan for your own future.

Grief takes time so be patient with yourself. Here are some things you can do as you reconcile your loss:

- Give yourself small rewards along the way and don't feel guilty about treating yourself to something.

- Take a short trip. Your grief will still be there when you return but you'll discover that you can still enjoy some things in life.

- Keep a journal. It is very therapeutic to write down your thoughts and feelings during this time.

- Plan ahead to deal with holidays and anniversaries. Don't wait until the last minute to prepare for those times. That empty chair at the dinner table can be celebrated with a toast, a prayer, flowers, and a photo of your loved one.

- Seek the comfort of your religious affiliation if you belong to a church group. Clergy, counselors, and support groups are there to help you. Even if you aren't a church member, there are grief support groups in your community that can provide an outlet for you to express your grief.

As the internal part of loss, grief is a process - a journey but with time, those open wounds will become scars and healing will take place.

Check It Out

Web Sites

- www.compassionatefriends.org

- www.DailyStrength.org

- www.From heartbreaktoHappiness.com

- www.griefjournal.com

- www.griefnet.org

- www.selfgrowth.com

- www.American hospice.org

Books

- *I Wasn't Ready to Say Goodbye: Surviving, Coping, and Healing After the Sudden Death of a Loved One* by Pamela D. Blair, PhD. & Brook Noel

- *Grieving the Loss of Someone You Love* by Raymond R. Mitsch & Lynn Brookside

- *When Bad Things Happen to Good People* by Harold S. Kushner

- *When You Lose a Loved One* by Charles L. Allen & Helen Steiner Rice

- *The Empty Chair* by Susan J. Zonnerkelt-Smeenge & Robert DeVreis

❦ *Part 5* ❦

Currency Considerations:
A Mini-Guide on Practical Matters

Does Money Make You Mean?

That question was posed by Jay MacDonald, a Bankrate.com contributing editor, in an article published on-line at AOL. He referred to a recent behavioral study that says people with money on their minds tend to be less helpful, less considerate, less willing to interact with others or even ask for help in completing a task. The findings were consistent in all nine experiments conducted.

Now while that type of behavior doesn't indicate being mean, it does illustrate that people in this category aren't exactly nice to be around. Well, what about you? What is your attitude toward money? In her book, *Build Your Money Muscles*, Joan Sotkin lays out two very important steps:

- preparing for financial change
- attaining a new financial identity

Her book will guide you through recognizing what she calls your "identity factor" which reflects your thoughts, beliefs, and feelings about money.

As someone who has "been there - done it" in terms of having experienced financial disaster, Sotkin is well-equipped to offer sound advice on how to understand the dynamics behind your current financial situation, raise your level of financial awareness, and set realistic goals for yourself. Her web site ProsperityPlace.com features articles, audio programs, e-books, and prosperity tips.

A study conducted for AARP Foundation's Women's Leadership Circle revealed that many women 45+ have a sense of false confidence when it comes to financial matters. While 61 percent of these women are confident that they will have enough money to enjoy life as they age, 62 per cent don't have a long-term spending plan for retirement. Two questions you need to ask yourself are:

- Do I have a financial plan?
- What will I be able to do in case of a financial emergency?

Does it surprise you to know that 80 to 90 percent of women will be solely responsible for their finances at some point in their lives? This high figure is due to divorce and widowhood since women outlive men by seven years.

Here are some interesting points to ponder:

- Sixty percent of America's wealth is controlled by women.
- Sixty-six per cent of women who work with a financial advisor feel more confident about having enough money in the future.
- Women retirees receive about half the average pension that men receive due to holding jobs that don't offer pensions or because they've changed jobs more frequently.

Here are some viable solutions:

- Check your investment accounts on a monthly basis to see if there any significant changes. You can do this when you're paying monthly bills.
- Don't be afraid to ask questions about risk, fees, and how the investment fits your strategy when you meet with your financial advisor.

- Stay updated in the financial markets and current economy.

Since women tend to reach retirement age with fewer resources than men, it means having less money which has to be stretched out over a longer period of time.

What Kind of Stool Are You Sitting On?

Barbara Kennelly, president of the National Committee to Preserve Social Security and Medicare, testified before the Senate Special Committee on Aging in March, 2006. She said that retirement used to be thought of as a three-legged stool. Social Security benefits, employer-sponsored pensions, and personal savings made up the legs. This has changed dramatically over recent years and now that stool can be compared to what she described as a "bar stool" with Social Security forming the central pillar upon which retirement rests. It is 52 percent of the total income for unmarried women over 65 and if it weren't for Social Security, two-thirds of elderly women would be impoverished. The two saving graces of Social Security are that the benefit lasts your entire lifetime and the Cost of Living Adjustment helps protect you against inflation.

On a more positive note, it may help to know that you may need less than you think for retirement. Except for healthcare costs which rise with age, there is a significant drop in spending in other areas by persons 65 and older. The figures released by the Bureau of Labor Statistics in 2005 show a 30 percent decrease in spending on housing, 42 percent for transportation, 34 percent for food and alcohol, 34 per cent for entertainment, and a whopping 46 per cent for apparel.

Meet Ms. Money

Well, her real name is Tiffany Bass Bukow but her web site, Ms.Money.com is another goodie you don't want to miss. You can brush up on the fundamentals of personal finance at the Beginner's Corner or check your money pulse in the Financial Health Section. You'll find great money-saving tips in her e-book *Live Your Life at Half the Price*. You can also visit the Women's Corner and take the Women's Money Seminar.

What Is Your Estate-Planning I.Q.?

Professional expertise on the subject of estate planning, trusts, and wills is readily available through seminars, books, and Internet. I would simply like to create an awareness and pique your curiosity to delve more deeply into this area.

Estate planning can be simple or complex, depending on your circumstances. It can be expensive or relatively cheap based on your worth; but having no plan at all is simply not a good idea.

Here are some options to compare and consider:

Trust vs. Will: A common will, also known as the Sweetheart Will, distributes all assets to the surviving spouse. If the total value of the couple's assets is under $2M (including life insurance) no estate taxes would be due upon the death of the surviving spouse. Two major drawbacks to this type of will are that it gives little protection to surviving children in the event that the surviving spouse re- marries or spends everything.

A complex will, on the other hand, directs assets ultimately to the children while providing a life estate for the surviving spouse.

A joint tenancy distribution can work well for a married couple who hold their property in this manner but it could create havoc for someone holding a joint tenancy with an irresponsible adult child. This can occur when people use joint tenancy for their home, automobile, checking and savings accounts.

Trusts come in all shapes and sizes. There are four good reasons for considering the creation of a trust:

- It avoids probate which can save time and legal fees since the assets are held in the name of a trust and not the individual.
- It helps minimize taxes.
- It provides on-going management of the estate to help insure that assets are invested properly
- Because it is a private document, no one can see it except the parties involved. Documents that go through probate are open to the public

Most banks and trust companies acting as trustees require that the trust be funded with at least $400,000 while others won't handle anything less than $1M.

Setting up a trust requires an attorney whose fees may range from $500 to $1500 for drafting the document. Handling fees vary.

Keep Your Eye on the Three Wise Men

Your financial advisor, broker, and elder lawyer should be looking out for your best interests. Don't take anything for granted. It's a good idea to maintain contact on a regular basis and double-check everything, no matter how sound the advice may seem. They may be well-intentioned but they are not infallible. If you do not engage the services of such persons, you can find valuable information at websites listed in the Check It Out section.

Insurance: A Quick Overview

- **Term insurance:** This type of insurance is meant to replace your income for any dependents left behind. Guess what? If you outlive the term of your insurance, you get nothing. A study done in the early 90's revealed that only one per cent of the 20,000 term policies reviewed in the study resulted in a death claim. Yet many people opt for this type of insurance because it is cheap.

- **Cash Value insurance:** This type of insurance allows you to accrue a cash value inside the policy which is somewhat like a savings account in addition to providing a death benefit. You may withdraw, borrow against, or leave the entire amount to your heirs. There are three major types: whole life, universal life, and variable life.

- **Long-Term Care:** If you haven't taken out this type of insurance by the time you're 40, you can expect to pay high premiums. If you have a policy and you want to keep it, Harry S. Margolis, an elder law attorney, suggests that you do one of two things - reduce the benefits to keep the premium the same or stop paying the premium and the insurer will pay claims in the future equal to the amount of premiums paid in to the account.

- **Short-Term Convalescent Care:** This type of insurance provides coverage for persons who may require home health care or adult day care services for a period of time but are expected to recover. There is also a plan that covers 30 days of inpatient care through a Hospice Care program.

- **Disability:** Most people don't think about insuring their careers. Since most baby boomers are continuing to work, it is probably a good idea to consider this type of coverage in the event you become disabled. The Health Industry Association of America claims that 30 per cent of Americans are likely to become disabled for at least 90 days. Workman's Compensation and Social Security won't necessarily meet your needs.

Suddenly a Widow: 9 Contacts You Need to Make

Losing your spouse plunges you into grief where even simple daily tasks become burdensome. Yet there are certain matters which must be taken care of immediately in order to protect your financial future. David W. Latko, president of Latko Wealth Management Ltd is the author of *Financial Strategies for Today's Widow* and he offers some sound advice:

- Obtain at least 10 certified copies of your spouse's death certificate from your local health department. You will need them to present to financial institutions and others. They will keep them for their records.

- Contact your spouse's former employer. When speaking with the benefit plan administrator, you will want to ask about any accrued but unpaid salary, sick leave and vacation days, commissions (if applicable), 401(k) accounts, and life insurance that your husband would have been entitled to receive. You must also decide if you want to continue health coverage if you had this insurance through your husband's employer.

- If your husband had life insurance, call the company that issued the policy. Latko recommends transferring the lump sum into a money market account until you're better able to decide on how to invest the money.

- Call the Social Security Administration (800-772-1213) or log on to www.ssa.gov/survivorplan/index/htm to notify them of your husband's death. You will receive his payments or your own - whichever is the greater amount - if you have reached 62. You will also receive a one-time $255 death benefit.

- Go to the bank or any other financial institution where you have accounts to change those accounts to your name only.

- Call the Motor Vehicle Administration to cancel your husband's license and arrange to have the titles on any vehicle to your name.

- Notify credit card companies, mortgage lenders and others regarding debts you held jointly with your husband. Ask if they have a record of any payment protection plan having been signed.

- If your husband was in the military or a veteran, contact the U.S. Dept. of Veteran Affairs (800-827-1000). You may be entitled to some benefits.

- Report any income your husband may have earned in the year of his death to the person who prepares your taxes. You can still file a joint return for the year in which your spouse died and claim deductions as long as you don't itemize.

Check It Out

Websites
- www.free-financial-advice.net

- www.americasaves.org

- www.fool.com/fa/finadvice.htm

- www.guardingourwealth.com

- www.moneywisewomen.net

Books
- *Becoming a Money Wi$e Woman: Getting Your Financial House in Order and It's All Fixable: A Woman's Guide to Managing Money & Creating a Healthy Financial Life* by Marcia Brixey. Order at www.cafepress.com

- *Financial Planning for Women* by Ernst &Young

- *Suddenly Single: Money Skills for Divorcees and Widows* by Kerry Hannon

- *It Takes Money, Honey* by Georgette Moshbacher

- *The 9 Steps to Financial Freedom* by Suze Orman

- *Build Your Money Muscles* by Joan Sotkin

Bargain or Wallet-Buster?

Shopping… at the mall, on the Internet, or by catalog is a tantalizing adventure that many women thoroughly enjoy. It can be disastrous for the women on a fixed income.

The majority of women entering the Age of Elegance don't have unlimited resources to indulge themselves with carefree shopping. Wealthy women aren't necessarily elegant just because they have more money to spend. One can exude elegance wearing thrift shop clothes if she knows how to pull it off. Good taste has nothing to do with how expensive something is.

Those catalogs that come in the mail can be real temptations to buy items one really doesn't need - be it clothing or household gizmos to make life easier. One little trick that works like a charm is to cut out the pages with items that appeal to you; clip them to the order form and then place them in your pending file for at least a week. That "cooling off" period will help you determine whether you really want or need those items.

Amazon.com allows you to place items in your Wish List. This way, you can put things on hold for a few days before placing them in your shopping cart. It is an excellent tool for self-control over what you spend. Shopping, like drugs and alcohol, can be an addiction for some women who seek to compensate for other things missing in their lives. If it is a serious problem for you, then seeing a counselor for help is something to consider.

More Savvy Shopping Strategies

When shopping at the supermarket -

- don't fall for those "Buy three for $5. Ask for the sale price for one item. You can still get the sale price for one at most stores.
- buy fruits in season or you'll be paying for transportation costs that have skyrocketed.
- just buy food. Period. Non-food items can be purchased elsewhere at much lower prices.
- avoid buying portion-controlled snacks. They are very expensive and you can make your own portions from a larger box using Ziploc bags,

- think twice about buying food enhanced with supplements. You'll save money by purchasing the same supplement in pill or capsule form.

When shopping for electronics-

- select a no-name brand. For cameras, DVDs, and TVs the difference in price is substantial while there is little difference in quality or performance.

- For more information on the different brands, log on to www.Cnet.com and click on "compare prices".

When shopping for clothing -

- don't thumb your nose at thrift shops or hospital shops run by the ladies' auxiliary. You can find quality clothing for a fraction of what you'll pay in department stores.

- visit the $15 Store at www.15dollarstore.com

Household Innovations for the Elegant Woman

The woman who has reached the Age of Elegance sees the wisdom of re-thinking her priorities. Household tasks and cooking, for most women, don't command their attention like they once did.

I have been known to post a sign on my front door from time to time which reads: "I cleaned my house last month - sorry you missed it!" This doesn't mean that I'm a slob. I keep a clutter-free, orderly home. I simply don't dust, vacuum, or scrub as frequently as I used to. Kitchen clean-up happens while I'm preparing food - not afterward. My bathroom gets cleaned when I go in to take a shower… and blessed is the person who came up with idea of those Clorox Handi-wipes!

Organized Elegance

Whether you live alone or with a partner, you can establish your residence as your elegant domain if you make a conscious effort to not just reduce - but abolish clutter. In the past couple of years, family and friends have enlisted my help in packing for a move to a new home. I tell them that the first order of business is to have three large, empty boxes in each room. They are labeled Pack, Discard (meaning give away or sell), and Undecided. If you begin in one corner of the room and work your way around, you'll be pleasantly surprised at how efficiently you work. While helping one friend, I discovered that she had thirty-nine boxes of tea in her kitchen cabinets and didn't have a clue that she had that many!

A couple of years ago, I decided to put my house up for sale. Within a few weeks, I had a contract with a prospective buyer and put a contract on a house I planned to buy but the contract on my house fell through which meant I had to withdraw the contract I had. Meanwhile I had already packed up everything except the bare bones necessities. Boxes, labeled and sealed, were stacked in my garage. Two bedroom closets were empty. Drawers and cabinets in the kitchen and dining room were bare except for essentials.

After recovering from the initial shock of what had happened, I abandoned the idea of moving but decided to leave things exactly as they were, figuring that if I should decide to move in the future, most of the work was already done. The playful side of me mused that if I should die in the meantime, my kids would have less to do. I discovered that I didn't need all that stuff after all. Packing away memorabilia, framed photographs, and other treasured items was actually quite easy because I know that the memories are very much alive within me.

Entertaining with Style

The Woman of Elegance is savvy about preparing food that is nutritious as well as pleasing to the eye. Whether cooking for company or just for herself, she adds those little touches that grace her table. Color, shape, and texture play an important role in her presentations. She doesn't agonize over menus because she has established a repertoire of luncheon and dinner entrees that have become her trademark.

The Woman of Elegance entertains graciously in a relaxed atmosphere because she plans dinner parties that don't require time in the kitchen after her guests have arrived. She wants to enjoy time with her guests. She selects dishes she can prepare in advance - a hearty turkey-ham-Swiss bake or a pasta casserole. Other vegetables can be micro waved in advance and re-heated before serving. Her guests will never see dirty pots and pans stacked in the kitchen sink.

Instead of serving a tossed salad, she places salad greens in a serving bowl and then arranges the other salad items in partitioned serving dishes so guests can choose what they want just like they do at a restaurant salad bar. Small bowls of soy nuts, sunflower seeds, and grated cheese add a nice touch. The Woman of Elegance never puts bottled dressings, ketchup, or mustard on the dining room table. Cruets or small glass bowls set on saucers will draw admiring glances from her guests.

She selects a wine that compliments the main course and may offer a liqueur like Amaretto with coffee after dinner. Desserts don't have to be made homemade or expensive to buy. I serve ice cream and cookies almost exclusively. I scoop ice cream into sherbet glasses and arrange three varieties of cookies around the edge of each glass.

With whatever table linens and dinnerware she has, the elegant woman knows how to embellish her table with carefully selected candles and flowers - and she never uses scented candles as it would throw off the odor and taste of what is being eaten.

Multi-tasking in the Kitchen: A Practical How-To

Multi-tasking is something women have done long before the word was ever coined but now the time has come to create a less demanding schedule and focus on the things you really want to do. This means spending less time in the kitchen. It can, however, lead to poor nutrition or relying on fast-food restaurant dinners loaded with calories and other harmful ingredients.

With careful planning, you can prepare four or five days' worth of dinners in less than an hour. They can be stored in your refrigerator or be frozen. Of course you can buy frozen dinners at the supermarket but aside from the expense, they contain high amounts of sodium and preservatives that may be hazardous to your health.

Here is a sample of a multi-tasking dinner preparation:

What you will need -
2 chicken breasts
2 pieces of fish
1 ½/c. each: pasta, rice
1 sweet potato
1 pkg. frozen vegetables

Place a pot of water to boil for pasta. Pre-heat oven or toaster oven for chicken and fish. While oven is heating, place rice in microwave to cook. While pasta and rice are cooking, prepare chicken and fish to bake or broil, using condiments of your choice. Place in oven. Pasta will require 12-15 minutes, depending on the type you select. Chicken and fish will require 20-25 minutes.

When rice is finished, place frozen vegetables in the microwave. Cooking time averages 5-7 minutes.

While the chicken and fish are still in the oven, the pasta should be ready to drain. It can then be placed in a covered plastic bowl filled with cold water until you're ready to use it.

The sweet potato can be micro-waved for approximately 8 minutes and later transferred to a toaster oven before serving.

Salad preparation can also be done in advance by using partitioned dishes or plastic containers for cut -up vegetables such as tomatoes, cucumbers, zucchini, peppers, mushrooms or anything else you wish to use. If you're not using bagged salad greens, heads of lettuce can be cleaned and stored in your vegetable bin. Lettuce leaves should be wrapped in paper towels and placed in a sealed plastic bag.

Clean-up time is snap if you clean as you go. Saving it for last defeats your purpose if you're striving for efficiency.

A Daily Dessert Loaded with Nutrition

What you will need:
1/2 banana (sliced)
1/2c low-fat yogurt
1 tsp. flax meal

Arrange fruit at bottom of cereal bowl. Sprinkle flax meal and wheat bran on top of fruit. Add yogurt, granola, and sliced almonds. You can substitute cranberries, diced dried apricots or strawberries. Delicious and non-fattening!

Bag It! Crate it! Put It in a Basket!

You can solve your storage problem simply and economically. Those haphazard closets and messy shelves can be eliminated completely and you can do it in no time at all.

First of all, take inventory of your needs. As you go from room to room, take note of what bothers you the most. Is it your kitchen cabinets where there is a jumble of canned goods, mismatched plastic containers, and condiments? Is it your hall closet where you see a tangled array of linens, towels, medicines, and personal hygiene items? If you keep gift wrap on hand, how is it that you never find it? And the bedroom closet? You don't even want to think about that one but you must!

So let's tackle the problem right now! Here are the tools you will need to get started:

- plastic shoe boxes with lids

- junior crates and mini-crates

- zip lock bags: gallon and quart -size

- plastic baskets: utility bins, under-the-shelf-baskets

- shelving space makers

- labels, tape, marking pen

Buy what you think you will need for the most troublesome area you want to tackle first. For example, in my kitchen I wound up using 14 junior crates, 3 small plastic baskets, and 1 plastic shoebox - all for under $20.00 at the dollar store.

Remember how your teacher made you categorize words when you were in the fourth grade? Put that skill to good use and categorize items on your shelves. Then crate and label them. The crates stack nicely on top of one another, creating even more space.

- A junior crate will hold 16 cans of pet food, 3 boxes of crackers, cookies or cereal bars, 9 large spice bottles, 6 cans of soup, or up to 6 bottles of vinegar, oil, gourmet sauce, and syrup. It is also good for storing soft packages of rice, beans, lentils and popcorn, opened bags of candy or chips.

- A covered plastic shoebox will hold 4 boxes of spaghetti, 12 pairs of pantyhose, 12 pairs of socks.

- A small plastic basket can hold up to 6-8 bottles of vitamins, 6 packages of Jell-O or pudding mix, 3 boxes of teabags (24count), 8 washcloths individually rolled, and up to 16 pairs of panties individually rolled.

Crates and plastic shoe boxes are perfect for the linen closet. For example, you can use the following categories: Cough and Cold, First Aid, Dental Care, Lotions, Hair Care.

- A silverware divider tray is equally good for holding pens, pencils, scissors, and a small stapler.
- Film containers make excellent storage for paper clips, thumb tacks, and safety pins.
- An assortment of wicker baskets in varying sizes can come in handy for storing pet grooming supplies, telephone books, and magazines.

Did you know that -

- empty baby wipes (the rectangular kind) are perfect for storing nail care items?
- an acrylic bagel holder for cutting holds 6 small bottles such as eye drops and nose drops?
- a child's plastic cup holds up to 6 small tubes of assorted ointments and antibiotic creams? It can also hold small scissors nail clippers, razor, and emery boards.
- a napkin holder can hold 6 packages of gravy mixes?
- an accordion file can be used to store packaged gift wrap for every occasion?
- a banker's box (found in office supply stores is perfect for holding handbags or hats?
- zip lock bags are great for storing greeting cards? You will have cards for each occasion at your fingertips if you sort the cards and label each bag: birthday, get well, sympathy, thank you, holiday, and special occasion.
- empty Clorox Wipes containers can hold magic markers and pens?

The rewards of organizing your stuff are quick retrieval, better use of available space, and keeping track of what you have on hand. So go ahead—get started! Who knows? You may come up with more clever ideas yourself.

Files You Shouldn't Be Without

The elegant woman lives the axiom: a place for everything and everything in its place. She refuses to succumb to frenzy and whining because she can't find things. Of course, there are those moments when one simply cannot remember where something is but those moments can be greatly reduced without a lot of effort.

A hanging file located near the telephone center allows you to have current records and other pertinent information handy for quick reference and follow-up. Files you may want to have are:

- Bills to pay
- Monthly expenses
- House data
- Upcoming events
- Pending
- Church/club/organization data
- Miscellaneous

These files should be checked and cleaned out on a monthly basis.

Recycle! Recycle!

Yes, you can -

- water your plants with left-over water from your pet's bowl
- re-use aluminum foil and plastic wrap more than once. Wipe clean, dry, and store on a paper cardboard roll saved from paper towels.
- use the paper napkins from the dinner table to wrap up the gunk in your kitchen sink.
- use that coffee filter more than once if you've only made 2-4 cups the first time.
- use that old toothbrush for small scrubbing
- rinse out those zip lock bags and re-use them.

Women's magazines and the Internet abound in time-saving tips and devices. This is simply meant to jump-start you into action with a gentle push in the right direction as you make your way into the Age of Elegance.

Part 6

At the Boarding Gate

"The most creative force in the world is a post-menopausal woman with zest."

~ Margaret Mead

Lost Your Zest? Get It Back!

Many years ago, I heard a sermon that focused on attitude. The part I especially remember dealt with how a person can greet a new day. One can say: "Good God! Morning! or "Good morning, God!" The latter appealed to me as a solid expression of a certain zest for life. Until then, I hadn't thought about whether this quality was apparent in my own life. Since then, I have become more aware of its presence, not only in my life but in the world at large.

Unlike patience, perseverance, and empathy, zest does not depend upon certain circumstances to induce it. It is free-form and uninhibited; suited to every moment and purpose. It is the "how" of intense, vigorous pursuit of what is at hand: challenging the uncharted sea or simply smelling the roses.

Zest is the hallmark of athletes and mystics; prophets and politicians.

It deals with the manner and intensity in which things are done. It is not confined to any particular ethnic group. Yet, there are groups who exhibit it with a particular flair. Consider the Greeks and their wild plate-smashing spectacles at a party. Plate-smashing for them is a fine indicator that a good time was had by all. Have you ever watched Polish youth as they stomp and shout through their endless polkas? Such revelry! Such gusto! Such zest!

Religion and history are studded with personalities who displayed zest. You can work your way through the Old Testament and David with his marvelous psalms to St. Francis of Assisi with his passionate Canticle to Brother Sun and find zest. Alexander the Great ruled with it. And what about the Vikings and Columbus? Surely they explored with it. Our Pilgrim Fathers, Revolutionary heroes, and western pioneers fashioned our country in a spirit of zest and passion for life.

Zest can be readily identified in theatrical productions. Who can forget the brawny, lusty Zorba in *Zorba the Greek* or Tevye in *Fiddler on the Roof* with his rendition of "To Life"?

The relish for life comes through in the paintings of such masters as Delacroix and Toulouse-Lautrec. Their style, color, and subject matter reflect a keen enjoyment of what they observed and perceived.

One's spiritual life can be lived with zest as well. That venerable Benedictine monk, Dom Hubert Van Zeller, had the formula for it in his book, *We Die Standing Up*.

Sports and zest are easily correlated. We see it on the tennis courts, on the football fields, and across the land with countless Little League players.

There is a myriad of musical compositions that must be played with zest: Italian tarantellas, Jewish horas, national anthems, and military marches.

The Madison Avenue guys and gals have cornered the market and popularized it in their commercials. The Pepsi generation drinks with it; Old Milwaukee Beer fans go whaling with it; and odor-conscious people shower with it.

Life without zest is drab and uninviting; with it, satisfying and colorful. Those persons who cultivate it are blessed with gratification in all that can be felt and accomplished in the daily celebration of life.

You as the Lebenskunstler

Hannelore Hahn, founder and executive director of the International Women Writers Guild, offers additional insight to the meaning of zest

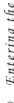

using the German word "lebenskunstler". In the December 2006 issue of the IWWG Journal, this is what she says: "Lebenskunstler […] connotes a person who approaches life with the zest and inspiration of an artist, although he or she may not be working recognizably as an artist. In other words, he or she may not be a painter or musician, but she approaches the canvas of her life with an impulse for self-expression and an intense desire to know, regardless of monetary reward. Furthermore, this attitude toward life is life-long. There is no built-in obsolescence. It makes for happiness and satisfaction throughout life and does not wear out until the body does. Her own inspirations, experimentations and devotions enliven her and others, regardless of age."

So listen to that inspirational voice deep inside you; be a risk-taker and experiment with something new; and define what you are truly passionate about and you will, indeed be a "lebenskunstler".

Do You Have a Ya-Ya Sisterhood?

When Rebecca Wells' best seller *Divine Secrets of the Ya-Ya Sisterhood* was first published, I scooped up a copy immediately. Hilarious, yet deeply moving, it is a story of life-long friendships and family loyalty. I could identify with the author because I, too, have been blessed with my own Ya-Ya sisters. We've been friends since second grade - spanning over 60 years. We've shared each other's joys and sorrows; confided in and sometimes even admonished one another. When the novel was made into a movie, the five of us went to see it, announcing to the theatre usher: "We ARE the Ya-Ya Sisterhood!" It turned out to be a memorable evening.

Even if your friendships don't go back that far, or time and distance have disrupted them, you can try to reconnect with the persons who have enriched your life in some way. My Ya-Ya sisters and I don't live near one another anymore but we schedule a time and a place to meet three or four times a year. It definitely adds zest to our lives.

Are You a Recess Girl?

Julie Lynn, a Play and Creativity coach, describes the Recess Girl as one who believes there needs to be more fun, play, and creativity in the world. She coaches women who want more fun in their lives; women who have dreams of finding their unique voice to express themselves creatively.

We can all remember recess as a very special part of our classroom day as kids. The child within us still begs to know if it's time for recess.

The woman entering the Age of Elegance allows herself "recess moments" because she realizes that it fosters healthy, vibrant aging. You can visit Julie at http://www.recessgirl.com to find out more.

Meek Little Lamb or Roaring Lioness?

Which one are you? There are so many older women who think of themselves as "invisible". Simply log on to numerous web sites where these support group discussions take place and you'll discover that an alarming number of women appear to have resigned themselves to the role of meek little lamb. Perhaps it's time to invite that roaring lioness within you to emerge, giving you the courage to explore your dreams and talents.

In her book, *Defying Gravity*, Prill Boyle tells the stories of 13 women, including herself, who as late bloomers, have "defied gravity" to listen to their hearts and follow their dreams. Sampling their stories is not only inspirational but essential for the woman who is timid about taking that first step.

Another must-read book that will help you in your quest to re-capture your zest is *Invisible No More* by Joyce Kramer, Renee Fisher and Jean Peelen. Their stories will also inspire you as you re-evaluate your life and ponder the endless possibilities that lie ahead.

Dawn Breslin, an internationally acclaimed self-development coach offers 10 dynamic life-changing solutions for self-empowerment in her book, *Zest for Life*. She describes it as a self-help bible and urges readers to read it once a year in order to review their self-beliefs and habits. There are exercises such as a self-expression checkup, vulnerability check, and identifying the toxic people in your life. Journaling topics are also available.

This book will help uncover what you believe about yourself; identify the things that you envision as an ideal life. Breslin's Five Magical Ingredients are powerful tools that you can use right away and she also provides four pages of ready-made affirmations to help you along the way.

Are You a Gutsy Woman Traveler?

Where in the world have you been? No, it isn't your mother asking you that - although you may have heard it from time to time after coming home a half - hour late from a date when you were a teenager.

Seriously, where in the world have you been? We're not talking business trips here. Many women travel as part of their jobs but that kind of travel leaves little or no time for exploring and submerging yourself in the local culture whether here or abroad.

For 40 years, I have traveled all over the world, defying the odds that I wouldn't be able to afford it or go it alone. I went solo on my first trip to Europe when I was in my late 20s and have traveled alone many times since.

My goal was to set foot on all 7 continents and I finally achieved it with a trip to Antarctica in 2005 - going solo once again because I couldn't convince any of my friends to join me. I figured that there would be another 199 people aboard the expedition ship so I wasn't going to be exactly alone. It turned out to be one of the most memorable trips I have ever taken. I met wonderful people from all over the world and was never at a loss for friendly conversation or table mates. I have traveled to the Middle East, South America, and New Zealand on my own recently and found the same camaraderie.

"But," you say: "I can't afford that kind of travel." With the exception of Antarctica which is somewhat pricey, I can tell you that the other trips were much less expensive than you would imagine. There are three rules I follow:

1. Book your own air travel and hotels.

2. Book your own daily sight-seeing excursions.

3. Nix the idea of a 5-star hotel and fancy restaurants

I don't go abroad to eat and sleep; I can do that perfectly well at home. I want to see and experience. I have feasted my eyes on the great works of the Masters in Europe;played with kangaroos in Australia's Outback; gone horse-back riding along the river in Christchurch, New Zealand; ridden a camel in Egypt; and danced on the Great Wall of China.

If the hotel is neat, clean, well-lit and in an area that is accessible to points of interest, that's all you need. There are many fine, low-cost restaurants everywhere but who says you have to eat out all the time? I love going to the local supermarkets or carry-out shops to pick up something for a meal to bring back to my hotel room. Many hotel rooms even have a kitchenette. After a full day of sight-seeing, there is nothing better than to sit back and relax with a glass of wine and "dinner" while watching something on TV.

A friend of mine recently widowed and in her early 70s, caused me to shriek with delight as she recounted her recent adventure in northern Canada. Dog-sledding had long been one of her dreams. She made that dream come true with an adventure expedition in Val-des-Lacs in Ontario. She not only mushed and tried ice-fishing; she slept in an Algonquin tent in the wilderness. Now that's zest at its best!

Pat Johnson and Regina Fraser, two middle-aged African-American women, are best friends who have traveled to over 80 countries over the past 30 years. Their focus is on tracking down cultural treasures, which led to a new TV series on PBS called "Grannies on Safari."

What I consider a primer for the older woman who wants to travel is the late Jay Ben-Lesser's book, *A Foxy Old Woman's Guide to Traveling Alone – Around Town and Around the World.* Her "Nine Steps to Confident Solo Travel and Tips for the Solo Traveler" will guide you every step of the way in planning your own travel adventure.

Check It Out
- www.journeywoman.com
- www.gutsywomentravel.com
- www.travelaloneandlikeit.com
- www.adventuredivas.com

Calling All Gorgeous Grandmas!

This wonderful concept originated with Alice Solomon shortly after her graduation from Wellesley College at age fifty. Alice re-entered the work world after many years of raising a family and became a syndicated newspaper columnist writing "A Guide for Gorgeous Grandmas". It has blossomed into radio and TV appearances, magazine articles, and her book, *Find the Love of Your Life after Fifty* published in 2004.

When you visit her web site, you'll be able to read the eight qualities she identifies as who the gorgeous Grandma is. My personal favorite is: "Loves life - and lets everyone know it!" Log on to http://www.gorgeousgrandma.com for a real treat.

Musings by Mekis

On a recent visit with a very dear friend of mine who spends part of the year in Florida to escape the harsh Maine winters, I was delighted to see how she had decorated her condo, giving it her unique signature in every room. What especially caught my eye and captivated me was what she did on one dining room wall. Helene wrote her ideas on life using every letter of the alphabet! Read and savor her thoughts:

Always avoid always.

Believe that you can.

Celebrate the beauty of diversity.

Dreams are for doing.

Enjoy the gift of each day.

Freak out a friend.

Give from the heart.

Humor gives perspective to life.

Intuition is a compass.

Jump at the chance to be playful.

Keep hope alive.

Laugh often to live well.

Make waves to float your boat.

Negotiate!

Open your mind to new things.

Perfection is highly overrated.

Quirky is interesting.

Read from the Book of Life.

Screw up -everyone else does!

Take the time to "BE".

Unleash kindness.

Vision helps one think outside the box.

Write love letters to loved ones.

Xpect the unexpected.

You-nique is what you are.

Zip through life at a snail's pace to savor it as you go.

When Was the Last Time?

When was the last time you -?

- relaxed in a warm bubble bath with scented candles and soothing music
- went for a long walk on the beach at sunrise
- spent the whole day doing absolutely nothing except reading and napping
- talked to your plants
- ate cold pizza for breakfast and bacon, eggs, and pancakes for dinner
- written a letter to the editor on an issue that concerns you
- fed the birds and squirrels in your backyard
- danced around the house alone to your favorite music
- spent an entire weekend with no radio, TV, or phone calls
- looked into the mirror and said:" Hey Kid, you're okay!"

A Little Zest Quiz

Have you ever-?

- gone "singing in the rain" like Gene Kelly
- stood outside howling at the full moon just for fun
- eaten dessert before dinner
- paid the toll for the person behind you at the tollbooth
- initiated a conversation with a stranger on the bus
- paid a compliment to the clerk at the checkout counter
- called the head honcho of a company to praise the service you received from one of his employees
- tried playing the harmonica or xylophone

A To Do List Worth Doing

- Send someone a lovely letter.
- Deliver a treat to your local fire fighters or sanitation crew.
- Get a Swedish massage.
- Join an art or yoga class.
- Forgive someone who needs your forgiveness
- Write down all the things you are grateful for.
- Volunteer at a homeless shelter, children's hospital or animal shelter.
- Limit your TV time and do something creative instead.

Please Remember Me!

If you were to write your own obituary, what would you want it to say? Everyone wants to be remembered for something. In an article entitled" Giving Back Is Food for the Soul", published on the Internet and adapted from his book *The Power Years: A User's Guide to the Rest of Your Life*, Ken Dychtwald asks some thought-provoking questions: "What will be your mission and your legacy? Will you make a mark or will you fade into a meaningless 'Jurassic Park' of unending play and self-absorption? Will you leave the planet having taken more than you have given? Will you use the gift of longevity to obsess about your wrinkles or rise to your greatest height?"

Your legacy will be something that can be preserved by future generations within your family or in the larger circle of the world you've lived in. Many people equate leaving a legacy with leaving large sums of money but that is a tiny part of the bigger picture. It can be concrete or abstract - ranging from an exquisite piece of jewelry to your philosophy of life.

When you create your legacy, you are, as Abigail Trafford says in her book, *My Time*, "giving a gift with a message. You want to speak to the next generation." George Vaillant describes you as "Keeper of the Meaning" in *Aging Well*, based on the Harvard Study of Adult Development.

Whether your legacy is public or private, it is up to you to begin the process while recognizing that you have no control over what will happen to it in the future. Think about the legacies that have been handed down to you - the customs, beliefs, ideas that have molded you and you begin to understand the generational transmission that keeps on flowing.

Not everyone is meant to accomplish grandiose projects that will affect the world at large but we can all do some soul-searching that will lead us in the direction of creating some small but significant contribution that will, in effect, be our legacy.

Find a Need and Fill It

Years ago when I first heard this statement quoted from an interview a reporter had done with A.G. Gaston, a prominent Black businessman who played a pioneering role in the South, I decided right then and there to make it my own philosophy of life.

Some forty years later, when I decided to enter the Ms. Maryland Senior America Pageant, one of the requirements was to give your philosophy of life within 45 seconds. I capitalized on that statement about find a need and fill it, using it in my presentation. Someone told me later that the impact of what I said on the judges scoring that day put me over the top. I won the title of Ms. Maryland Senior America 2003.

So where do you begin? Outside the circle of your immediate and extended family, opportunities abound. What are the requirements? A generous, compassionate heart, the gift of your time, and the willingness to put your best talents to work as a volunteer are all that you need. Here is a short list of organizations you can check out for further information:

- **USA Freedom Corps:** supports Federal service programs; serves as a resource for non-profits; helps to connect individuals with volunteer organizations in their communities. For more information, call 1-877-872-2677 or log on to www.USAFreedomCorps.org.

- **Senior Corps:** helps volunteers to serve through the Foster Grandparent, RSVP and Senior Companion programs. For more information, call 1-800-424-8867 or log on to www.seniorcorps.org.

- **Alternatives to Violence Project (AVP):** trains volunteers to conduct conflict resolution workshops in communities, schools, prisons, halfway houses, and women's shelters. For more information, call toll-free 1-877-926-8287 or e-mail avp@avpusa.org

- **Legacy Leadership Institute:** recruits, screens, trains, and places volunteers in civic engagement in public policy, nonprofit fundraising, humor practices, environment, health and independent living. For more information, call the University of MD Center on Aging at 301-405-2470.

- **AARP:** works closely with community partners to ensure that AARP programs are available in their community. Volunteers help with a variety of community events. For more information, call 1-888-687-2277.

- **S.C.O.R.E. :** uses volunteers to counsel thousands of small business owners and entrepreneurs from nearly 400 offices nationwide. For more information, call 1-800-634-0245.

- **Peace Corps:** serves 73 countries world-wide, using the skills and life experiences of volunteers in programs covering education, health, environment, community development, and information technology. For more information, call 1-800-424-8580 or log on to www.peacecorps.gov.

How About a Senior-Friendly Volunteer Vacation?

Transitions Abroad offers an inviting spectrum of opportunities to vacation overseas and volunteer at the same time. Here is a sampling of what you may want to consider:

- **Earthwatch Institute:** an international nonprofit organization that places volunteers around the world with a menu of scientific and social science research. For more information, call 1-800-776-0188 or log on to www.earthwatch.org.

- **Habitat for Humanity:** an ecumenical Christian nonprofit organization that invites volunteers to help eliminate poverty housing around the world. No building experience is necessary. For more information, call 1-800-HABITAT or log on to www.habitat.org.

- **Global Citizen's Network**: a volunteer organization for people who are interested in sharing values of peace, justice, tolerance, cross-cultural understanding and global cooperation. For more information, call 1-800-644-9292 or log on to www.globalcitizens.org.

- **Oceanic Society Expeditions:** This nonprofit organization works to protect marine wildlife and environment. Volunteers work side by side with academic and field researchers, logging, recording and collecting data in the Central and South America and Pacific Ocean regions. For more information, call 1-800-326-7491 or log on to www.Oceanic-Society.org.

- **Orphanage Outreach:** an interdenominational nonprofit organization that supports orphanages in the Dominican Republic. Volunteers work with children educationally or on projects to enhance the orphanage facilities. For more information, call 602-375-2900 or log on to www.orphanage-outreach.org.

Research shows that persons who have a higher level of education, who are religiously active, and in good health are more likely to volunteer. It also found they like to be asked personally, favor a short duration of time, and prefer flexibility in scheduling their volunteer hours. But please! Don't wait to be asked - find a need and fill it. Whether you help out with Meals on Wheels, coach a youth group in sports or the arts, visit an elderly person who never gets a visitor, help other seniors prepare their tax returns, or cuddle a sick baby in a hospital, you will be, in effect, establishing your legacy for your family's future generations.

Everything I know about selfless giving, I learned from my grandmother and my mother. I can still remember accompanying my grandmother as a youngster to Ft. Meade to visit the Italian prisoners of war. Her legacy to us was a deeper understanding of compassion. Tears still well up in my eyes when I remember how my dear mother, desperately in need of a new winter coat, went without in order to buy us a set of encyclopedias that year. Her legacy to us was that of life-long learning and personal development.

Most women I've spoken with say they want to be remembered for being there when needed or being faithful but there are a number of women out there who, as one woman put it, "don't have a clue." Let's hope that that you're not one of them.

So there it is…pure and simple. Getting involved, giving back is a way to pursue your passion and nourish your soul while leaving a legacy that is meaningful and worthwhile.

Check It Out
- www.legacymemoirs.com
- www.lifeinlegacy.com
- www.getinvolved.gov

Think MSN

No, it isn't the Microsoft Network I'm talking about here. I'm offering you a little mnemonic device to help you remember three important words -

mentoring, supporting and networking. As you enter the Age of Elegance, these areas can and should have a special place in your life.

No matter what your situation is, staying connected is essential to living a life that you deserve. The Woman of Elegance is aware of the importance of "being in touch". She doesn't pursue meaningless, trivial matters just to fill in the time. She surrounds herself with people and activities that nurture her. This includes social, volunteer, political, and spiritual contacts which allow her to remain vibrant, engaged, and interesting. She is also aware of the necessity of having a solid support system for problems which may arise from time to time.

You as a Mentor

Your accumulated wisdom gathered through the years can provide help to younger women in so many ways. Whether your expertise comes from having a degree in a particular field or was acquired through the School of Hard Knocks, you surely have something to offer.

A mentor advises guides, supports, tutors, and coaches. First and foremost, she is a role model and she knows how to listen. By sharing her strengths, she becomes stronger.

There are so many young women who could use your help: in schools, prisons, abused women's shelters, and perhaps even in your own neighborhood. Mentoring can help them face daily challenges; stay focused, and improve their attitude.

Women in business are especially interested in having an informal mentor - someone they can turn to for consultation about their careers. The Simmons School of Management conducted a survey revealing these facts:

- 82% of business women have an informal mentor.
- 60% report that their mentors are female whereas in the mid-1990's only 17% of mentors were female.
- 77% of the women surveyed serve as mentors themselves.

Mentoring involves trust and a safe place to express one's concerns. The mentor can provide invaluable help with information and resources, guidance in exploring options, and support that the younger person needs as she considers her possibilities for a satisfying, productive life.

Become a Mommy Mentor Partner

Mommy Mentors began in 2004 as a resource for all women, regardless of age, marital status, motherhood or not. This women's on-line community will help you to find and offer support with daily issues ranging from simple to complex. There are articles to read and interviews with experts to listen to plus a message board where you can chat with other members.

Using the power of their own real life experiences, Mommy Mentor partners give hope and inspiration to those who need it. Family, motherhood, friendship: these are the ideas that Mommy Mentors holds sacred. Log on to www.mommymentors.com for further information.

Beyond Support Pantyhose

"Nothing beats a great pair of L'eggs". The Hanesbrands Inc. was right on the money with that catchy logo. Most of us have worn support pantyhose to help with swollen ankles or aching legs - not to mention the benefits of moderate support to the tummy and thighs.

Support… Roget's Thesaurus lists more than twenty synonyms for this word and the three words I would like you to consider go beyond support pantyhose. These words are: sustain, shoulder, bolster. They can be used to describe what a good support group can do for someone reaching out for help.

There are support groups for all types of health issues and personal challenges. You can meet with a support group within your community or join a support group online.

The Woman of Elegance handles adversity with dignity and grace but she is also wise enough to know that she may need some help along the way. Support groups exist to help people who are in similar situations. By sharing their concerns with one another, they also learn from one another

When looking for a support group, there are several things you should consider:

- How much of yourself are you willing to share? Support groups are not appropriate for everyone. In some cases they might actually add to one's stress rather than relieve it.
- What is the nature of your need? Severe psychological or marital problems are best handled through individual counseling with a licensed clinical social worker or therapist.

- Are you looking for a professional group leader or someone "who's been there - done that" experience? How upset are you? If you're feeling too distressed, it might be better to wait until you're feeling less anxious. Listening to other people's problems might be too much to handle and you're not likely to benefit from the group in that state. When selecting a support group, be aware of some dos and don'ts:

DO find out:

- the history of the group and how stable it is
- the mix of the group. Is there a good balance between members who have been there for a while and newcomers?
- how the leader operates. Is that person capable of drawing out shy members and tactfully keep others from dominating the discussion?

DON'T join a group that -

- conducts gripe sessions.
- recommends a single solution to a problem.
- pressures members to buy certain products.
- charges high fees. Most support groups are free or collect voluntary donations. Others may charge a small membership fee to cover the cost of handouts or refreshments.

There are many fine support groups everywhere. Obviously they cannot all be listed here but as befits the nature of this book, I want to mention SOWN which fits into the categories of support and networking.

SOWN, the acronym for Supportive Older Women's Network was launched in 1982 by Merle Drake. It began in Philadelphia but has since grown to over 80 local and 47 national support groups serving over 3,000 older women.

New program and services continue to be implemented. In addition to support groups, SOWN offers workshops, counseling services, and training programs which address the specific concerns of older women. They also collaborate with leading universities in conducting extensive research relating to issues older women face. Their motto is: SOWN… because no woman should have to age alone. For more information, call 215-477-6000 or e-mail: info@sown.org. Their web site is www.sown.org.

Another impressive source for information on support groups is Daily Strength. You will find 500+ support groups listed on their web site. Doug Hirsch, Josh DeFord, and Lars Nilsen are Internet veterans with plenty of experience at building and running Yahoo Groups and GeoCities. They invite supporters and medical professionals as well as those who need a helping hand. You can check out all the support groups from A to Z as well as information on doctors and treatments by logging on to: http://www.dailystrength.org.

Just Heard It Through the Grapevine!

Networking goes far beyond the business world and today's women have harnessed it to broaden their world. There are many women's networks to choose from, depending on your interests or needs. As you enter the Age of Elegance, you may want to explore some of the organizations listed here. Most women do have a healthy social network consisting of family and friends but it is equally important to develop an expanded network related to who you are at this point in your life.

Since we are living in the Cyber Age, a great deal of networking takes place on the Internet. You can, however, connect with other women in these organizations through local chapters that host breakfasts and dinner meetings, teleseminars, and workshops.

FYI: The organizations featured here are but a sampling of what is available but they represent a nice variety of options you can consider so go ahead and explore!

National Association of Baby Boomer Women

NABBW is the front-runner organization addressing issues concerning 38 million Boomer women who are "the healthiest, wealthiest, best-educated women ever to hit mid-life" according to Dotsie Bregel, founder and president.

Together with its sister site, www.boomerwomenspeak.com, NABBW is dedicated to empowering women to explore their passions and live life to the fullest. You'll find expert advice on everything from Empty Nest to Fearless Aging. Women who are still working can access a wealth of information ranging from Winning at Work to Web Site Development. Visit NABBW's web site at www.nabbw.com.to read the Top Ten Things Boomer Women Want in 2007 or e-mail: info@nabbw.com. Membership is $75 annually.

Boomer Babes Rock!

Allison Bottke, a Christian writer and founder of this web site says: "The hubris of youth is behind us and the wisdom of the years has made us pretty darn attractive - both inside and out." On this premise, the Boomer Babes Rock web site will guide you to turning your dreams into realities. You can download free inspirational messages, participate in teleseminars and check out Boomer Babe Bloggers. You can also subscribe to DreamZine where you'll find resources and tools to help you achieve your goals. DreamZine is sent via e-mail on the third Wednesday of each month. Allison also hosts godallowsuturns.com and has authored 21 books.

For more information, log on to www.boomerbabesrock.com or call 507-334-6464.

Vivacity

If you're asking yourself "What's next in my life?" check out http://www.vivacity.com. This multimedia information center offers services and products to help every woman answer this question. Membership is free and training, guidance programs and networking opportunities are available in person, by phone, and on- line. Kate Sanner, founder and CEO of Vivacity can be reached at 1-888-285-4038 or e-mail: kate@vivacitynow.com

Black Women's Network

This network provides a forum for learning, enrichment, encouragement and support for black women worldwide. Founded in 1997, Black Living grew out of an awareness that the concerns of black women were not addressed adequately.

The web site features expert advice and ideas on everything from health and beauty to careers and money. Gloria Sawyers is the founder and publisher of Black Living. For more information, log on to www.blackwomensnetwork.net .

Powerful You!

This organization was founded on the belief that women are powerful creators, passionate and compassionate leaders; the heart and backbone of the world's businesses, homes, and communities. It welcomes women from all walks of life who want to connect and grow in their business and personal relationships. It offers local, live chapter meetings nationwide as well as telenetwork meetings. There is an annual membership fee of $125. The cost for Tele-network membership is $75 annually. Contact Sue Urda or Kathy Fowler at 973-248-1262 or e-mail info@PowerfulYou.com.

Older Women's League

OWL is the only national membership organization dedicated to address-ing the needs of mid-life and older women. It works to create a level playing field so that women have the resources and opportunities they need as they grow older.

Pivotal issues for OWL include long-term care, mental health, public transportation and America's retirement system as it pertains to women of diverse communities, particularly African-American, Asian-American and Hispanic women.

Through grassroots education, advocacy, and media campaigns, OWL works on issues of importance to older women. For more information call the OWL Powerline at 800-825-3695 or log on to www.owl-national.org.

Gather the Women.org

This web site serves as an interactive communication hub for women around the world. Using the Internet as a global communication tool, over 4,700 women from 67 countries have connected with one another in their shared vision of activating the power of women's wisdom on a planetary scale.

GTW was launched without funding and no brochure has ever been printed; yet it continues to grow. For more information e-mail: info@gath-erthewomen.org.or call 949-454-1349.

Fifty and Furthermore.com

Dr. Dorree Lynn, psychologist, media expert, and author of *Getting Sane without Going Crazy*, hosts this web site where you can find information on topics ranging from mental health to sex over 50. There is even a page on career/ reFIREment. Click "On the Couch with Dr.Dorree Lynn". There you can read articles like "Breaking Bad Habits (and learning which ones to keep)" posted by Dr. Lynn. Her latest book, *When the Man You Love Is Ill: Doing Your Best for Your Partner without Losing Yourself,* offers practical, compassionate advice to women who face the challenge of caring for a seriously ill husband.

Foundation for Conscious Evolution

Here is another source that addresses change in the global context. Its vi-sion and goal is to awaken the spiritual, social, and scientific potential of humanity in harmony with nature in order to achieve the highest good of all life.

Through education and networking FCE is helping to build what they term "a golden bridge" to the next stage of evolution - a future free from illness, hunger and war. For more information visit www.BarbaraMarx-Hubbard.com or www.Evolve.org.

Evolutionary Women.org

This organization is dedicated to making women visible to each other and the world as the new Feminine Archetype of the 21st Century through events, retreats, forums and teleforums. Evolutionary Women has created a vehicle for women to connect and explore how to use their talents, skills, and presence to contribute to the evolution of humanity, with a vision for a world of peace and justice.

Lucky Sweeny and Bonnie Kelly are the co-founders of Evolutionary Women with years of coaching experience between them. For more information visit www.Evolutionary Women.org or e-mail: info@evolutionary-women.org.

AuthenticWoman .com

Minx Boren, BA, PCC and Marsha Lehman, M.Ed, RSP.are dedicated to bringing women together through ritual, play, deep discussion and conversation that celebrate the feminine spirit. If you're ready for a new beginning - with your health, relationships, soul, perhaps even a second career, check out Fresh Start. You'll also be able to participate in telebridge calls featuring topics like Pleasurable Practices vs. Dreary Disciplines. There is much more including a CD entitled "Getting in Touch with Your Inner Coach" as well as books that will capture your imagination. For more information log on to: www.authenticwoman.com

Refugee Women's Network

This national non-profit organization, created in 1995, focuses on enhancing refugee and immigrant women's strengths, skills, and courage. It offers leader ship training, education and advocacy to promote independence and self-sufficiency among its participants. RWN is governed and staffed by refugee and immigrant women from Africa, Asia, Europe, the Middle East, and the Americas.

Through its leadership training program, over 300 women in 30 states from over 40 countries of origin have graduated. In Atlanta, GA, RWN is helping women start, expand or strengthen their business through its micro loan program which has a zero default rate.

The National Conference of Refugee and Immigrant Women provides hundreds of women with the opportunity to learn new skills and learn from each other. For more information log on to www.riwn.org or e-mail: director@riwn.org.

Code Pink

This grassroots peace and social justice movement works to end all wars and re-direct resources into education, healthcare, and other life-affirming activities. Its creative campaigns began in 2002 when co-founders Medea Benjamin, Jodie Evans, Starhawk, Diane Wilson, and Gael Murphy took to the streets of Washington, D.C. with approximately 100 other women and set up a four- month vigil in front of the White House to protest the Iraq War. Now there are over 250 active local groups around the country and the world. Code Pink women have also traveled to Iraq, Afghanistan, Jordan, and Iran to deliver humanitarian aid and establish diplomatic and human connections.

Regional offices are located in Los Angeles, San Francisco, Washington, D.C. and New York City. For more information log on to: www.codepink.org.

Women of Color Network (WOCN)

In 1997, a group of women of color banded together to provide leadership and resources to promote the activities of women of color advocates and activists. They also have an active Mentor Project assisting close to 300 women across the United States and Territories. WOCN is a project of the National Resources Center on Domestic Violence but leadership, staff, and WOCN advisors are made up exclusively of women of color.

There are two levels of membership: Patron at $30 annually and Sterling at $50 annually. WOCN also has a scholarship and financial assistance fund.

WOCN publishes Voices twice a year. Their "Facts & Stats Collection" provides excellent information on sexual violence and domestic violence as they relate to:

- African-American women
- Asian and Pacific Islander women
- Hispanic/Latino women

- Native American and Alaskan Indian women

For more information contact WOCN at 800-537-2238 or e-mail: wocn@pcadv.org . Their web site is www.womenofcolornetwork.org.

Red Hat Society

This group began in 1998 with Sue Ellen Cooper's impulsive purchase of a red fedora at a thrift shop. The rest is history. It is the result of a few women deciding to meet middle age with verve, humor, and élan. After shouldering responsibility at home and in the community for many years, they decided that it was time "to do for themselves".

The Red Hat Society originally described itself as a "disorganization", as it doesn't have rules or by-laws. Instead, it focuses on enabling its members (approaching the age of 50 and beyond) to connect with like-minded women in search of fun, friendship, freedom and self-fulfillment. Garbed in purple dresses (inspired by Jenny Joseph's poem "Warning") and red hats, they meet in local chapters in all 50 states as well as 28 other countries. For more information call 714-738-0001 or log on to: www.redhatsociety.com.

The Global Goddess.com

Similar to My Space, You Tube and Facebook, this web site provides members with the opportunity to connect with friends and business associates. Photo slide shows, video players, music players and network badges can be embedded anywhere on the Internet, thus funneling new people into your network. To make new friends and business contacts, log on to www.theglobalgoddess.com.

Women & Hope

By sharing resources, knowledge and inspirational stories that will motivate women to live their dreams, this web site offers support, advice and encouragement to women world-wide. Members can add a profile, list events to the calendar, add photos and participate in discussion forums. For more information, log on to: http://womenandhope.collectivix.com or e-mail Dr. Deitra Payne at drcami2@cs.com

EMwomen

Staci Wallace, nationally acclaimed motivational speaker, author and life coach founded EMwomen with the commitment to educate and empower women to make the best decisions in the areas of family, finance, fitness and faith. There are many groups to choose from in the EM community. For more information, log on to: http://.emwomen.ning.com or e-mail info@emwomen.com.

As you enter the Age of Elegance, you may be experiencing menopause or have already gone through it. That means you're ready for what Barbara Marx Hubbard calls "regenopause - the pause in the life cycle of the older woman when the possibility of remaking herself by choosing from her deepest impulse becomes evident."

By channeling your passions, creativity, and dreams through one of the resources listed here, you have the opportunity to enhance your life and to be a role model for younger women as well. So go ahead... explore and enjoy!

❧ *Part 7* ❧

Ready to Fly?

A Little Homework Assignment

At the beginning of this book I asked you to do several things:

- take an inventory
- reflect on packing for a journey
- consider yourself as a debutante
- explore the meaning for rite of passage

As you read through each section, you either came across information you already know or discovered something that you didn't know.

Many educators guide their students through the K-W-L process: what I <u>K</u>now about this topic; what I <u>W</u>ant to find out; and what I have <u>L</u>earned as a result of reading about this topic. Even without knowing the K-W-L process, you most likely did the first two steps subconsciously when you first picked up the book. Now I suggest that you consciously complete the third step. Write down at least 5 new pieces of information or ideas that you feel you have learned.

Your second assignment is this: create your very own rite of passage ritual. Here are the basics:

- Find a quiet spot in your home or garden.
- Arrange flowers and candles on a table
- Select some lovely background music to play.
- Read aloud any passage or poem that you feel is appropriate for the occasion.
- Spend a few minutes in total silence and reflection. Think about all that you've witnessed and experienced in your lifetime. Give thanks for all the good memories you have. Feel the magic of what lies ahead.
- Now celebrate with your favorite dessert!

Carefully Chosen Words

I didn't feel that this book would be complete without mentioning three pieces of writing that I personally treasure. These writings reflect in some way what I have attempted to convey throughout this book. One is written by one of the most elegant women I know - poet Maya Angelou. In *Phenomenal Woman*, she speaks about the "grace of my style" and not having to "shout, jump, or talk real loud" in order to be noticed.

The second piece, one attributed to the Dalai Lama, offers sage advice such as "Take into account that great love and great achievements involve great risk." There are a number of web sites which post *Instructions for Life* where you can read the entire piece. It is probably a condensed version of a Nepali Good Luck Tantra Totem associated with an ASCII art representation in 1999.

Finally, Frank Kaiser, a writer and host at www.SuddenlySenior.com has this to say about older women:

Frank Kaiser on Older Women

As I grow in age, I value women who are over 40 most of all. Here are just a few reasons why: A woman over 40 will never wake you in the middle of the night to ask, "What are you thinking?" She doesn't care what you think.

If a woman over 40 doesn't want to watch the game, she doesn't sit around whining about it. She does something she wants to do. And it's usually something more interesting.

A woman over 40 knows herself well enough to be assured in who she is, what she is, what she wants and from whom. Few women past the age of 40 give a damn what you might think about her or what she's doing.

Women over 40 are dignified. They seldom have a screaming match with you at the opera or in the middle of an expensive restaurant. Of course, if you deserve it, they won't hesitate to shoot you if they think they can get away with it.

Older women are generous with praise, often undeserved. They know what it's like to be unappreciated.

Women get psychic as they age. You never have to confess your sins to a woman over 40. They always know.

A woman over 40 looks good wearing bright red lipstick. This is not true of younger women or drag queens.

Once you get past a wrinkle or two, a woman over 40 is far sexier than her younger counterpart.

Older women are forthright and honest. They'll tell you right off you are a jerk if you are acting like one. You don't ever have to wonder where you stand with her.

Yes, we praise women over 40 for a multitude of reasons. Unfortunately, it's not always reciprocal. For every stunning, smart, well-coiffed, hot woman of 40+, there is a bald, paunchy relic in yellow pants making a fool of himself with some 22-year-old waitress.

Ladies, I apologize for all of us.

Last Minute Details

So... now it's time to check out a few things for that fabulous journey you are about to make. There are four things you must have in your possession if you're ready to fly – and I hope you are!

Check Your Luggage

The seasoned traveler knows the importance of listing all the items she will need to pack so as not to forget anything. Leaving needed items behind only creates frustration and unnecessary expense. Your list for this incredible journey into the Age of Elegance should include the following:

- Values, virtues, and qualities you wish to personify.
- Experiences that you find fulfilling.
- At least 10 things you hope to accomplish with the rest of your life.
- People and events that make you feel more alive.
- Talents which you have and can use to make a difference.

Your Itinerary

A well-planned itinerary includes a day-by-day synopsis of the places you will visit, hotel accommodations, land travel arrangements as well as arrival and departure schedules.

Your itinerary for this special journey should include:

- contacts you can make - some of the organizations mentioned in this book
- books you want to explore further as a result of reading this book
- web sites you plan to check out
- quotations you want to remember
- affirmations you plan to use
- a short-term/long-term plan of action

Print Out Your Boarding Pass

Thanks to the Internet, travelers now have the option of printing out a boarding pass 24 hours prior to a scheduled flight, thus saving time having to wait in line at the airport. Your boarding pass for this journey should include the following information:

- Destination: the Age of Elegance

- Date of Departure: Now

- Departure Gate: Discovering my vital, self-affirmed, authentic Self

Your Passport

A U.S. passport contains your photo, name, sex, birthplace, birth date, nationality, issue date and expiration date. It is considered property of the U.S. government and must be surrendered upon demand made by an authorized agent of the State Department. It is not valid unless signed by the bearer. The passport is stamped upon entry and departure from the country one visits at the airport's immigration checkpoint. The first page of the passport reads:

"The Secretary of State of the United States of America hereby requests all whom it may concern to permit the citizen/national of the United States named herein to pass without delay or hindrance and in case of need to give all lawful aid and protection."

So now, dear Lady, consider this:

Your passport has been issued for travel into the Age of Elegance; to pass "without delay or hindrance" into a world full of new beginnings and adventure; a world where you will be given the opportunity to make wise, elegant choices; a new frontier where you will invest your time and energy in a self-defining mode on things that matter to you the most.

Are you ready? Bon Voyage!

Litany of Elegance

Blessed is the woman who affirms herself each day

Blessed is the woman who believes that beauty comes from within.

Blessed is the woman who challenges media stereotypes of aging.

Blessed is the woman who dares to try something new after fifty.

Blessed is the woman who envisions change as an opportunity.

Blessed is the woman who focuses on the "bigger picture" - not just herself.

Blessed is the woman who grants herself permission to make mistakes.

Blessed is the woman who handles adversity with dignity and grace.

Blessed is the woman who initiates dialogue with her younger counterparts.

Blessed is the woman who joins a group trying to make a difference.

Blessed is the woman who knows the difference between aggression and assertiveness.

Blessed is the woman who learns the difference between sex and love.

Blessed is the woman who manages her money wisely.

Blessed is the woman who nurtures the young with her wisdom and experience.

Blessed is the woman who opens her heart to the less fortunate.

Blessed is the woman who prioritizes her needs with integrity.

Blessed is the woman who questions The Establishment when she sees immorality.

Blessed is the woman who relishes her role as mentor and legacy leader.

Blessed is the woman who speaks with quiet authority.

Blessed is the woman who trusts her instincts on when to act.

Blessed is the woman who understands that aging gracefully is something to be proud of.

Blessed is the woman who values her own worth.

Blessed is the woman who wears her silver hair and wrinkles like a badge of honor.

Blessed is the woman who opts to X out negative thinking.

Blessed is the woman who yearns for that which is substantial and not superficial.

Blessed is the woman who zeroes in on the qualities that will help her become ...

A Woman of Elegance

~ Chloe Jon Paul

Elegance Showcase: 20 WOW Women

Maya Angelou	*Poet, Author*
Brooke Astor	*Socialite, Benefactress*
Ingrid Bergman	*Actress*
Roselyn Carter	*First Lady*
Joyce Clautice	*Ms. Senior America 1999*
Candy Crowley	*CNN White House reporter*
Princess Diana	*English Royalty*
Ruth Bell Graham	*Wife of evangelist Billy Graham*
Ellen Sirleaf Johnson	*President of Liberia*
Coretta Scott King	*Civil rights activist, wife of M. L. King*
Wilma Mankiller	*First woman chief of the Cherokee Nation*
Patsy Takamoto Mink	*First Asian-American congresswoman*
Helen Mirren	*Actress*
Marily Mondejar	*President of Filipina Women's Network*
Toni Morrison	*Winner of Nobel Prize in literature*
Jacqueline Kennedy Onassis	*First Lady*
Eleanor Roosevelt	*First Lady*
Beverly Sills	*Opera star*
Meryl Streep	*Actress*
Oprah Winfrey	*TV personality, humanitarian*

These women were chosen because they each exemplify a certain type of elegance that I admire. Now...who would be on your WOW list? Why?

Epilogue: After All Is Said and Done

Now that you have "boarded your flight" into the Age of Elegance, please give your undivided attention to the following "flight instructions" to insure a safe, pleasant journey.

A wise Indian guru once described humans as being a house with four rooms: the physical, mental, emotional, and spiritual. He said that we tend to spend most of our time in only one of those rooms and that it would be in our best interests to visit each room daily.

While reading this book, you had the opportunity to explore each of those "rooms". Hopefully, this allowed you to decide how to tackle what needs refurbishing and repair. This leads to thinking about how to make elegant choices. In her book, *Elegant Choices, Healing Choices*, Marsha Sinetar explains that "elegant choices are those options that are, by and large, tending toward truth, beauty, honor, courage – choices that are life-supporting both in motive and quality. Elegant choice is neither stylish nor trendy."

Remember how we used to refer to the main subjects taught in school as the 3 R's? Well, now you have another set of 3 R's to think about: reflect, resolve, regenerate.

- Reflect on what you have read and develop an action plan.

- Resolve to put your action plan to work immediately and aim for consistency.

- Regenerate into the vibrant, graceful, elegant person you were meant to be.

Have a fabulous trip!

Bibliography

Angelou, Maya. *Phenomenal Woman: Four Poems Celebrating Women*. New York: Random House, 1994.

Barr, Karen. *For My Next Act*. New York: Rodale Press, 2004.

Ben-Lesser, Jay. *A Foxy Old Woman's Guide to Traveling Alone*. Freedom, CA: The Crossing Press, 1995.

Berkewitz, Bob. *What Men Won't Tell You But Women Need to Know*. New York: Avon Books, 2005.

Blair, Pamela D. PhD. *The Next Fifty Years: A Guide for Women at Midlife and Beyond*. Charlottesville: Hampton Roads Publishing, 2003

Blair, Pamela D. Ph D.and Brook Noel. *I Wasn't Ready to Say Goodbye: Surviving, Coping and Healing After the Sudden Death of a Loved One*. Naperville, IL: Sourcebooks, Inc., 2008

Bolen, Jean Shinoda, M.D. *Crones Don't Whine*. Boston: Conari Press, 2003

Borysenko, Joan. *A Woman's Book of Life* .New York: Rivermead Books, 1998

Boyle, Prill. *Defying Gravity*. Cincinnati: Emmis Books, 2004

Brady, Shelly. *Ten Things I Learned from Bill Porter*. Novato, CA. New World Library, 2002

Breathnach, Sara Ban. *Something More: Excavating Your Authentic Self*. New York: Warner Books, 1998

Breslin, Dawn. *Zest for Life*. Carlsbad, CA: Hay House Inc., 2004

Bridges, William. *Managing Transitions: Making Sense of Life's Changes*. Cambridge: DeCapo Books, 2004

Canfield, Jack & Mark Victor Hansen, *Chicken Soup for the Soul*. Deerfield Beach, FL: Health Communications Inc., 1993.

Chodron, Pema. *When Things Fall Apart*. Boston: Shambala, 1997

Chopra, Deepak. *The Seven Spiritual Laws of Success*. San Rafael: Amber-Allen Publishing, 1993.

Coelho, Paulo. *The Alchemist*. San Francisco: Harper, 1993.

Cooper, Sue Ellen. *The Red Hat Society*. New York: Warner Books, 2004

Crisp, Wendy Reid. *100 Things I'm Not Going to Do Now That I'm Over 50*. New York: Perigee Books, 1995

Culbreth, Judson. *Boomer's Guide to Online Dating*. New York: Rodale, 2005

Curry, H., Clifford, D. & Frederick Hertz. *A Legal Guide for Lesbians & Gay Couples*. Berkeley: Nolo Press, 2005

Doress-Worters, Paula B. & Diana Siegal Laskin *Ourselves, Growing Older*. New York: Simon & Schuster, 1994

Dychtwald, Ken & Daniel J. Kadlec. *The Power Years: A User's Guide to the Rest of Your Life*. Hoboken: John Wiley & Sons, 2005

Egoscue, Pete. *Pain Free for Women*. New York: Bantam Books, 2003

Ellison, Sheila. Ed. *If Women Ruled the World*. San Francisco: Inner Ocean Publishing Inc., 2004

Falk, Florence. *On My Own: the Art of Being a Woman Alone*. New York: Harmony Books, 2007

Godden, Rumer. *A House With Four Rooms*. 1st ed. New York: William Morrow, 1989.

Goleman, Daniel. *Emotional Intelligence*. New York: Bantam, 1995

Goldman, Caren. *Healing Words for the Body, Mind and Spirit.* New York: Avalon, 2001

Gray, John. *Men, Women and Relationships.* New York: Harper Paperbacks 1993

Gunn, Timothy. *A Guide to Quality, Taste, & Style.* New York: Harry N. Abrams, 2007

Hannon, Kerry. *Suddenly Single: Money Skills for Divorcees and Widows.* New York: John Wiley & Sons, Inc., 1998

Hyman, Mark. Dr. *Ultrametabolism.* New York: Scribner, 2006

Jacobs, Ruth Harriet. *Be an Outrageous Older Woman.* New York: Harper Perennial, 1997

Janis, Martin A. *The Joys of Aging.* Dallas: Word Publishing, 1998

Keith, Jon. *Everyday Memory Builder.* New York: Bookspan, 2006

Kramer, J., R.Fisher, and J. Pielen. *Invisible No More.* New York: IUniverse Inc., 2005

Ibid. *ABC's for Seniors.* Greentop, MO: Hatala Geroproducts, 2006

Kreamer, Anne. *Going Gray: What I Learned About Beauty, Sex, Work, Motherhood, Authenticity & Everything Else That Really Matters.* New York: Little, Brown & Co., 2007

Kushner, Harold. S. *When All You've Ever Wanted Isn't Enough.* New York: Summit Books, 1986

Ibid. *Living a Life That Matters.* New York: Anchor Books, 2002

Latko, David. *Financial Strategies for Today's Widow.* New York: Simon & Schuster, 2003

Levine, Suzanne Braun. *Inventing the Rest of Our Lives.* New York: Viking, 2005

Lynn, Dorree PhD. *Getting Sane Without Going Crazy.* Philadelphia: Xlibris, 2000

McClelland, Carol L. *The Seasons of Change.* Berkeley: Conari Press, 1998

McFarland, Judy L. *Aging Without Growing Old.* Palos Verdes: Western Front Ltd., 1997

McHugh, Mary. *How Not to Become a Little Old Lady.* Kansas City: Andrews McMiel Publishers, 2002

Ming-Dao, Deng. *Everyday Tao.* San Francisco: Harper, 1996

Patterson, Kerry et al. *Crucial Conversations.* New York: McGraw-Hill, 2002

Peck, Scott. The Road Less Traveled. NY Simon & Schuster 1993

Rountree, Cathleen. *On Women Turning Forty.* Freedom, CA: The Crossing Press, 1991

Rowe, John W. & Robert L Kahn. *Successful Aging.* New York: Dell, 1998

Sinetar, Marsha. *Don't Call Me Old! I'm Just Awakening.* New York: Paulist Press, 2002

Ibid. *Elegant Choices, Healing Choices.* New York: Paulist Press, 1988

Small, Gary. *The Memory Bible.* New York: Hyperion Press, 2003
Ibid. *The Longevity Bible.* New York: Hyperion Press, 2006

Snowdon, David. *Aging with Grace.* New York: Bantam, 2001

Solomon, Alice. *Find the Love of Your Life After Fifty.* Cranston: The Writers Collective, 2004

Sotkin, Joan. *Build Your Money Muscles.* Santa Fe: Prosperity Place Inc., 2006

Spezzano, Chuck. *If It Hurts, It Isn't Love.* New York: Marlowe & Co,.1998

Sultenfuss, Sherry & G. Thomas. *A Woman's Guide to Vitamins, Minerals and Alternative Healing.* Chicago: Contemporary Books, 1999

Tessaro, Kathleen. *Elegance.* New York: William Morrow, 2003

Trafford, Abigail. *My Time.* New York: Basic Books, 2004

Vaillant, George. *Aging Well.* New York: Little & Brown, 2002

Viorst, Judith. *Suddenly Sixty.* New York: Simon & Schuster, 2000

Ibid. *Necessary Losses.* New York: Simon & Schuster Fireside Edition, 1998

Vreeland, Diana. *DV.* New York: DeCapo Press, 1997

Warren, Rick. *The Purpose Driven Life.* Grand Rapids: Zondervan, 2002

Wells, Rebecca. *Divine Secrets of the Ya-Ya Sisterhood.* New York: Harper Collins, 1996

Wilson, Laura B. & Sharon P Simson Ed. *Civic Engagement and the Baby Boomer Generation.* New York: Haworth Press, 2006

Winter, Susan & Felicia Briggs, *Older Women, Younger Men: New Options for Love and Romance.* Far Hills: New Horizon Press, 2000

Von Zeller, Dom Hubert. *We Die Standing Up.* New York: Sheed & Ward, 1949

Other Media Sources

Available on CD

DeFoore, William PhD. "Elegant Aging: Growing Deeper, Stronger and Wiser in Your Years." Halcyon Life Enterprises, 2007.

Magazine Articles

Abram, Marjory. "How to Remove Personal Information from the Web". Bottom Line, Feb15, 2007

Desai, Roger. "Women & Investing: Take Control of Your Financial Life". Women's Journal, Feb/Mar 2006.

Dreifus, Claudia. "The Big Idea!" AARP, March/April 2006

Hubbard, Barbara Marx. "Regenopause". On Purpose Woman, Mar/Apr 2006.

Latko. David W. "Financial Steps After a Spouse Dies". Bottom Line, Apr.15, 2007.

Springen, Karen. "No Lift for Face-Lifts". Newsweek, March3, 2006.

Streisand, Betsy. "Turn Back the Clock!" US News & World Report, Nov.14, 2005

Website Articles

Davis-Ryzycki, Karla. "How to be Classy and Elegant without Money". http://www.ezinearticles.com.

Emotions Anonymous. "Helpful Concepts of the EA Program". http://www.emotionsanonymous.org.

Harper Collins. "Conversation with Kathleen Tessaro". June 2006. http://www.harpercollins.com.html

Hinderliter, Lynn. "Detoxification." http://www.vitaminlady.com/articles/detoxfasting.asp.

Howard, Caroline. "Goodbye to Hair Dye". http://www.coaches.aol.com/wellness/anne-kreamer. Accessed Oct. 23, 2007.

Kullander, James. "Turning Toward Pain: Interview with Pema Chodron." reprinted from The Sun magazine http://www.beliefnet.comstory/160/story_16054.hmtl.

Livini, Eprat. "Medical Science Meets Spirituality". http://.abcnews.gp.com/Health

MacDonald, Jay. "Does Money Make You Mean?" http://www.bankrate.com/brm/news/pf20070123_money_psych_al.asp.

Nelson, Mariah Burton. "Ageism and Aging Up". http://www.mariahburtonnelson.com./articles/Aging Article.

Redd, Nancy. "Over Fifty Fashion Tips". http://www.shoppingAOL.com/articles2008/04/41 what-not-to-.

Scholten, Amy. "How Stressed Are You?" http://www.beliefnet.com/healthandhealing/getcontent.aspx?c.

Van Mater, Ingrid. "The Mystery of Death and Rebirth". http://www.theosophy-nw.org/theonw/death.

About the Author

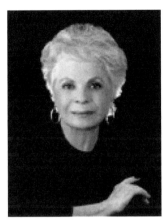

Chloe Jon Paul, M.Ed., is a retired educator and writer of several published articles and a book entitled What Happens Next: A Family Guide to Nursing Home Visits… and More.

Her many achievements include:
- Title of Ms. Maryland Senior America 2003
- Recipient of the Fulbright Fellowship Seminars Abroad award to South Africa, 1996
- Volunteer internship during the 2005 Maryland legislative session as a Legacy Leadership Institute graduate
- Lead facilitator for the Alternatives to Violence Project in prison and community workshops on conflict resolution for ten years
- State representative for the National Family Caregivers Association's caregiver community action network 2006-2008
- Advisory board member: MD, Healthcare Commission and the Interagency Commission for Aging Services: Maryland Dept. of Aging
- Hospice and homeless shelter volunteer
- Coordinator for the Good Samaritan Project at her church
- World traveler – all 7 continents

Chloe's philosophy of life is: find a need and fill it. She is the proud mother of son, Dominic and daughter, Alessa. Her 3 grandsons are her greatest joy. Chloe resides in Bowie, MD.